MITOCHONDRIAL MURDER?

POTENTIALS AND PROTOCOLS IN THE MITIGATION OF RNA BIO WEAPONS' EFFECTS ON THE HUMAN VASCULAR SYSTEM.

By Deirdre McNamara, D.Hom

Nothing "lab" proven, no experiments, funded or made. Just experience in the deeply researched, time honored, exceptional protocols of Homeopathy and logical analyses re the use of proven "externals." In brief, no fauci-faustus "clinical trials!"

Dr. Deirdre McNamara

drdhom@proton.me

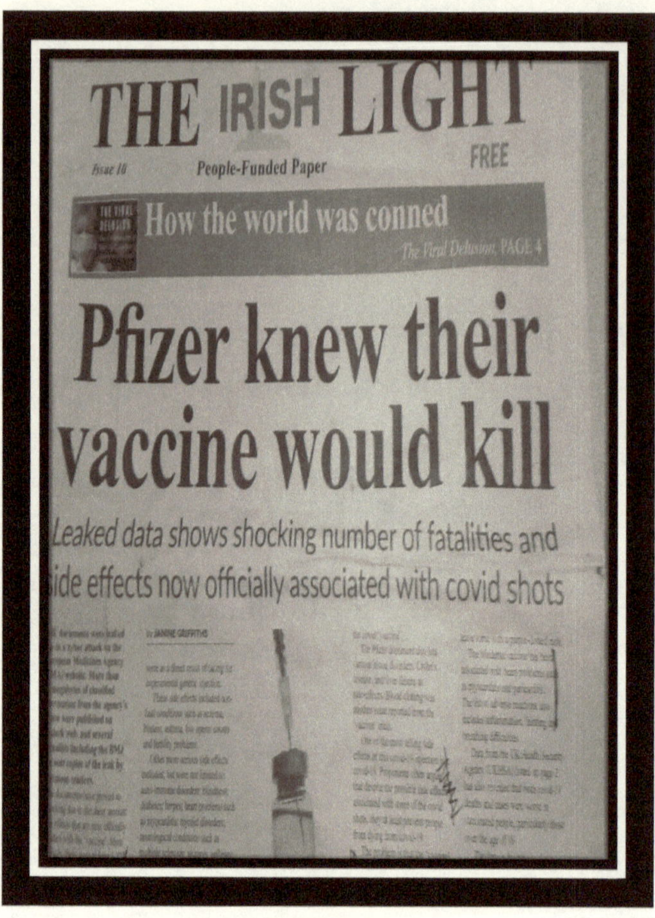

1,223 deaths in the first 28 days following shot...Prior to the Covid scandal, PFIZER had already sustained a *record* *$40 billion* in fines for: **false claims, med equipment safety violations; off-label promotions corrupt practices, kickbacks and bribery.**

https://phmpt.org/pfizers-documents

(Post marketing experience, 5.3.6)

"There is a lot of "it was the hit to his chest" that caused the American football player to collapse with a heart attack after the but look at rugby players, they're not padded up to the eyeballs and they take hits that would knock us ordinary folk out. The bottom line is...I was an athlete a sprinter in what they call now 100 metres sprint, in my day it was the 100 yards dash which is longer and I can tell you when I lined up my adrenaline was pumping which it had to as that is one's 'flight or fight' signal from the brain. Once that flag went down I was off running at high speed, I could actually feel my heart pumping blood around my body, after crossing the finishing line it was bend down, draw big breaths to get that air I had expelled back into my lungs, a few minutes and I was good to go. Not once in my day did any of us go down with any issue. The same with basketball, tennis, volleyball which I played: no issues. If people cannot connect the dots by now there is no hope for them going forward." Jan 4, 2023, Mrs. Maureen O'Leary

Maureen O'Leary is a member of Ireland's alternate media and frequent radio pundit.

Books by Deirdre McNamara and Donna Brava

HOMEOPATHY IN THE TIME OF COVID
HEART OF MERCY
PEPPERPOT POETRY: BANGOR TO BEYONDER
THE TUSCANY EXPRESS (Homeopathy. "ER")
CHILD SEXUAL ABUSE: NEVER CALL IT LOVE
THE SANITY OF CHRIST vs THE FALLACIES OF FREUD
SOS – FOR SURVIVORS OF SUICIDES
A WHISPER OF ANGELS

TRIBE OF CANNIBALS (The NY Gulag)
NEW CHRISTMAS STORIES – FOR CHILDREN OF ALL AGES (Fiction)
THE DEMISE OF SENATOR DUFF (Fiction)
THE FAMINE REPORT (Drama)

Other works of Fiction and Drama are archived in the National Library of Ireland and the Library of Congress, USA.

Original music manuscripts may be lost for ever along with many original dramas.

No rodents, mammals, bunnies, kittens, puppies, guinea pigs or other small creatures were tortured, maimed, harmed or killed in the foundational provings of Homeopathy, nor subsequently, nor in studies relative to the writing of this book.

We are not Pfizer. No "Fauci-Faustus" clinical trials.

Just deeply researched information and knowledge that has been proven to be precise, correct and profoundly effective for over two centuries; so effective, in fact, that millions of dollars were spent to suppress Homeopathy in the early and mid-twentieth century - by closing our Hospitals, University faculties, denying our physicians status, and failed at that, to complete distort our image and capabilities.

Prior to this, Medical and Life Insurers in the USA offered our patients discounts. It was well established that the patients of Homeopaths enjoyed longer life-spans with fewer illnesses, etc.

Surgeons at London's "Hospital for Special Surgery" requested our service prior and post procedure, because patients recovered faster, with fewer, if any, complications.

Homeopathy, correctly used, and with the full co-operation of the patient has cured: antibiotic resistant infections, infections, weaned patients off respirators, stopped cardiac arrests in progress, cholecystitis, infertility, etc., etc., asthma, allergies, post thrombosis paralysis, post traumatic paralyses, etc.

The Homeopath treats the patient, not the ICD code.

INDEX

Dedicated to those who stood for Truth and to those
bereaved by lies.

1. Retrospective. Time of Covid
October 2019 to Jan 2020

<u>Proning:</u>

Contra indicated in respiratory infections or afflictions eg   injury or post op. Blocks action of the diaphragm – ie the "bellows" or pump that opens and closes the lungs.

I would hold to this even if the entire corrupted element of the AMA claims otherwise.

<u>Paralysis</u>

New York Hospitals ran out of paralysands during the first promoted phase of the "Pandemic."

Proning + Paralysands = facilitating the "harvesting" or more precisely, "seizure of organs from living patients," a practice imported from China, doubtless by Fauci *et pals*.

The patient is immobilized by paralyzing drugs, but not anaesthetized. S/he is then placed face down, and the organs are removed, one by one, by one, the heart being the last to maintain maximum "freshness."

Despite declarations to family and friends that the patient is "brain dead," most patients are fully aware, and many weep through the procedure though unable to call out or move to defend themselves in any way.

Until proven otherwise, Fauci's intense relationship with China and his cold cynicism and facile lying in the White House Press Room makes him the most likely suspect for importing a system that horrified the world when imposed on political prisoners in China.

Or the front man for a massive, globalist cartel intent on depopulating the world and "keeping the land and venison" for itself and offspring. But what happens when there are no more people lining up to "buy diamonds" on the 13th of February each year...?[i]

Once NY ran out of paralysands, it was impossible to retrieve the living organs from still living patients, hence the return of patients to Nursing Homes and the people were waking up!

This was also contemporaneous to health professionals, such as myself, raising red flags and notifying the White House of the appearance of State sanctioned mass murder.

For this I may have lost my apartment in PA. The Chief "Health Officer" at the time was Dr. Richard-Rachel Levine, a psychiatrist apparently confused about gender, his own or others, or who just simply changed identity to avoid litigation relative to his "work" with vulnerable children in a NY residential home for minors with eating disorders.

NYPD cold case please investigate.

Corrupt MDJ James Gallagher unlawfully and illegally evicted me from my apartment, not only refusing to see proof of perjury by my opponent, but, in addition, ordered all reference to said proof wiped out, and, violating Federal, State and Local Laws, knowingly forced me into a nomadic lifestyle for almost three years. That is how corrupt and desperate the pHARMaceutical and government traitors were to keep the truth about "Covid" and the lethal injections from the public.

<u>Ventilators</u> **Lo-flo oxygen is comforting and helpful to patients with pneumonia, pleurisy, asthma and idiopathic forms of dyspnea. Oxygen pushed at high pressure into Remdesivir compromised lungs bursts the alveoli, causing the**

patient to drown in his/her own blood and pulmonary fluids. Death by lung puncture. In other words – AGONY.

There are rumors of individuals going through CV19 units, turning the vents up to the max, as many nurses refused to do so. As these were usually the nurses who refused the "clot shot" aka "vaccines," aka bioweapons, they lost their jobs. Not their lives nor their souls, however.

This was never the intention of President Trump!

Italian, American and Canadian doctors performing covert autopsies state that the lungs of the deceased Covid patients, ie, those who died in the hospitals, are punctured. They have "giant" holes. That, I interpret, is due to the ventilators set to the max. Remdesivir damages kidneys, damaged kidneys cannot filter urine and protect lungs, damaged lungs become oedematous and vulnerable, like soggy sponges.

High pressure ventilators may have their uses, but *never on highly compromised lungs...*

Protocols used for protection and contagion containment were hopelessly inadequate, and, in my professional opinion, valued or not, are tantamount to **reckless endangerment, manslaughter, or, if intentional, MURDER.***

Operation Paperclip,[1] anyone?

***Addendum April 20, 2023 - https://rumble.com/v2ip9c0-shocking-testimony-from-two-canadian-funeral-industry-professionals.html**

From New York City to Pennsylvania, Canada, Ireland, London, Italy, senior citizens were rushed to hospitals on the slightest pretext.

These so called "patients" remained isolated and unprotected in these so called hospitals and health care facilities until the Remdesivir ("kidney killer") provided them with the rationale for murder.

What did these senior citizens have in common?

They were "baby boomers," post war citizens determined that Nazi Germany would never happen again. They were witnesses, observers, heroic

---

[1] Post WWII, the US Government under Truman, imported Nazi scientist, giving them full status and access to laboratories and equipment. Might explain why Werner von Brauns rockets kept exploding. Most favored were biochemists working with the Pharmaceutical industry, eg, Bayer, Pfizer, etc., in Germany.

veterans, bereaved parents, widows, children, and even grandparents who survived the terrible wars.

The other factor was that these "baby boomers" were determined to work hard, acquire their own homestead and build a nest egg for their senior years, for emergencies, and for a "parting gift" for their children.

The deep state can print money. But they cannot expand the world's acreage.

The Creator can, of course, should He choose, but the cartels behind the Fake "pandemic" and the lethal "vaccines" are panicking as the world's population appears to grow, and so attempting depopulation on an unprecedented scale.

The "Covid" scandal was one continuous land and asset grab. I shall repeat this, *ad nauseum,* until the world awakens and screams: "No more political-medical MURDER," and "Stop taxpayer funding of private corporations."

I wrote to President Trump three times on this. He eventually "got the message," but by that time it was too late for his political career and for those who died.

The nation was in mourning. Mourning in lockdown. Lockdown so that they could not exchange information, compare notes.

15 minute cities are the latest extension on that.

2. COVID 19 – LIES, DAMN LIES AND STATISTICS!

Once upon a time, well after there "were wolves in Wales," and long after the "birds in red flannel petticoats"[2] had flown the "harp shaped hills"[3] and become "cardinals" in the Colonies, there were "Cowboys and indians." Then political correctness gave us "good sheriffs" and "Bad Barts."

Because Bolsheviks flooded into the USA, disguised as poor, pathetic refugees, systematically usurped the educational system, and imposed communist neo feudalism on the hearts and minds of our children – in addition to terrorizing the authentic refugees from Soviet Communism.

Suddenly, race and class divisions were institutionalised, "busing" became mandatory for grade schoolers with no consideration for the safety and comfort of each, individual child.

"One plus one" no longer equaled two, and a long series of "words, words, words"[4] and euphemistically termed "strings" replaced numbers and confused our children. Computation became an exasperating narrative of anomalous, polysyllabic word strings. Deborah Birx is an outstanding example of its mind numbing effects as she clenches her fists, Pelosi-Clinton style, and reiterates misappropriated polysyllables such as "granulation" for

---

[2] Dylan Thomas: "A Child's Christmas in Wales."
[3] ibid
[4] Hamlet by W.Shakespeare

charts and diagrams which show nothing of the true effects of induced disease progression or consequential human suffering.

For me, Birx is forever associated with the term: "Lies, damned lies and statistics"- statistics useless for the care and treatment of the suffering but essential for the tracking of the "failed" CV19, to ensure that CV 2020 came to full bloom just in time for maximum political damage on Nov 3, 2020.

I will never understand how President Trump did not fight the lies from the start. Surely he had met enough charlatans in New York City to recognise a scam when he encountered one.

Math is its own language: unique, direct and highly informative, it does not need an awkward and portentious patois. But we already know that. Speaking French, English, German and Italian simultaneously or in rapid sequence might be fun for a while, but is not recommended as a method of instruction and results in gibberish.

"Gibberish" is derived from "gibbet" or apparatus from which humans were once hanged. A "flibberdigibbet" was an evil spirit who flew by the gibbets seeking to capture the dying souls and take them directly to hell. Gibberish may be the language of the terrified, or the language of the dark side. Where Birx, Fauxci, Redfield and Hahn's "sound and fury signifying nothing" is concerned, the "dark side" seems to be the most likely source.

Unlike the UK where creativity and independent thought was encouraged, the NY Public School teachers found a way to make discovery and education an onerous, punitive, exercise in conditioning children to fill out forms and "just follow orders," and, through "book reports," destroy the joy of reading in small children. This transformation was instigated by the Bolsheviks who infiltrated the USA disguised as "refugees."

Does this sound familiar? Oh yes, there were thousands of authentic refugees escaping from the cruel Bolsheviks led by Vladimir Illych Lenin and cohort Stalin, but also thousands of "infiltrators," allegedly including the forebears of Obama's sponsors the Pritzkers. These were committed Communist scions from the USSR who faked refugee status in order to infiltrate and overthrow the United States of America through the educational system.[5] Their offspring lied[6] to the people of America in order to put the Communist Obama in the White House and paid his "stipend" for his fake job at U Chicago.

"Bad Bart" suddenly became the "good guy," the *victim*, and the "Good Sheriff" was now the villain. How *dare* he love his country, his constitution, history, traditions, family and law and order! And shock, horror, dismay, the Good Sheriff carried a *gun!*

---

[5] The late, great Fr Cosgrove, SJ, had an eidetic memory and recalled every action, every step, school, college, person and traitor in that system. He was not vindictive but deeply and appropriately concerned. Even "Ivy Leagues" have fallen under deep state control.
[6] Reliable, protected sources claim that the Pritzkers paid Obama's "salary" in U.Chicago as he was unqualified to teach or work there.

"Bad Bart's" guns are ignored along with every incendiary item including words and ideology! Arm the criminals, traitors and covert Bolsheviks.

Keep the people on edge, with a series of crises, followed by resolution. So the terrified people become the *grateful* people. Straight out of the "How to control your spouse: the Abusive spouses Handbook – political edition!" The dramas and crises are exhausting, so eventually the voter/victim says "leave them to it, I'm ok with Stockholm Syndrome," albeit secretly hoping for a rescue, a "savior." And "resolution" becomes regulation, and regulation, oppression! As the abused spouse dies silently, withering on the vine, so to speak, so also dies the nation!

However, when the Good Sheriff comes into town, takes out the bad guys, makes the streets safe for work, for leisure, for enterprise and brings it all back to life, the "Good Sheriff" is not immediately welcomed. The "Good Sheriff" is met with suspicion, even disdain: "Where were you when the attack came?" "Why didn't you speak up?" It is "irrelevant" that the "Good Sheriff" was himself or herself under fire, blockaded, injured.

It is far more comfortable to blame the outsider, the newcomer, the unknown, secret benefactor than to take responsibility for one's own naivete, or even stupidity.

Few men thrive in solitude. There are more monastics living in community than hermits, living alone, for example. Man does better in community, tribe, family and normally avoids ostracism, social isolation; is very slow to "rock the boat" and challenge authority; works well in teams. In other words, his nature is essentially *social.*

"*Socially,*" however, more objections to the 'scamdemic," masks, isolation, untested "vaccines" were initially raised by women. The men were mostly willing to "take one for the team!"

By all logic and reason, the manner in which vents were used on compromised patients appears to be the cause of far more fatalities than the "Covid virus"/flu 2019 vaccinosis itself.

To maintain the "reign of terror," a patient would be admitted with, say, an infected toe, immediately vented, prepped for surgery, and being diabetic, subject to further "infection," then the entire foot is amputated, followed the leg, and of course the diagnoses of Covid and the pressured oxygen., soon thereafter, a subsequent death cert of "death with Covid."

One of *thousands,* killed to divide, terrify and control.

All during this period, no physical contact with family was allowed. He had a cell phone that the nurses couldn't bothered recharging, etc., etc.

In the meantime, hypoxia inducing masks became pathogen producing mini "labs," and Heaven knows

what microbes were exhaled directly into the facial
orifices or nasal labia of the naïve and compliant.

There is no rationale for those danged masks, and
there are other, far more expedient and effective
means of containing *genuine epidemics*.

> *When the people start to cheer,*
> *Enter "Bad Bart," with a mask and sneer.*
> *The weak shiver and cower in fear –*
> *And blame the **Good** Sheriff.*
> *And so, to show "Bad Bart" they're on his side,*
> *They wear a mask and leer and jeer.*
> *Imprison children, and*
> *Plant their roadblocks everywhere*
> *While pilots die mid-air and cars collide...*

©2020 Deirdre McNamara

3.PUNITIVE PROTOCOLS

Proning patients with any form of respiratory distresses from colds, to flu, to asthma, to pneumonia, pleurisy, pleuro-pneumonia, sinusitis, etc., is obstructive, vicious and sadistic. Sedating or paralyzing such patients is not only cruel and obstructive but downright dangerous.

Placing a patient with respiratory challenges face down obstructs the movement of the diaphragm.[7] This inhibits respiration, is agonisingly painful and places him/her at high risk of thrombosis – even without the accursed mRNA - and, sudden death.

Prescribing renal compromising, kidney destroying Remdesivir to a patient with a diagnosis of "flu," which primarily affects respiration, is tantamount to cold blooded murder. Whether diagnoses were true or falsified. For mercenary purposes or in error.

It now appears that most diagnoses were falsified.

For mercenary purposes of hospital and medical practitioners, and the "deep state" depopulation agendae evident in CDC-WHO support of Big pHARMa, all of whom enjoyed billion dollar increases in income. The most lucrative mass murder in history.

Damaged kidneys cannot filter fluids and eliminate them...so the tissues bloat, becoming o/edematous -

---

[7] A "bellows" type muscle regulating the movement of the lungs.

swollen, soggy, the lungs like *sodden wet sponges, the alveoli saturated with fluid, leaving little or no room for oxygen absorption and easy targets for the highly pressurised bullets of concentrated air.*

Pushing pressurized oxygen into these "wet sponge" damaged lungs is insanity – unless the *intention* is death, in which case it is **homicid**e. Although inferior to Homeopathy, "Antagonistic" aka standard medicine has other beneficial, or less damaging protocols, not utilised and apparently not even considered!

Then again, what are the ICD codes for murder/manslaughter by Oxygen RX!

Nolle prosequi!

So it would appear that the mortality or death of their patients was the goal. At $50,000 per completed corpse, plus whatever they could get for remaining organs or bodies for "Anatomy 101" in med schools around the world, the "covid 19" genocide generated billions for all participating hospitals.[iii]

In addition to which, Deep State or rogue elements may have the intent or ability to seize assets, land, property, etc., because *Senior Citizens were the target. A bankrupt or greedy Government apparatchik would not turn down the death taxes and cessation of Social Security, etc.*

Adult children of bankers attended my former University: one the more frequent refrains in their confirmation was the "land" per se was the only asset that could never increase and therefore became more valuable over time. I often think of those comments now.

Senior citizens, i.e., the "boomers," the wartime and post war babies, who, determined to create a better world, saved, bought property, a little land, a home for themselves and their family...

It is for that very reason that they were targeted. Also because they are easy to scare into taking the "flu shots."

Despite the fact, that by self-definition, "Senior Citizens" must have sturdy immune systems, or they would all have died off before the first "Social Security" cheque.

So Seniors are not easy to kill naturally, but are holding on to land and assets not only envied by some, but deeply coveted, it would appear, by the deep state.

The speed at which NY Hospitals ran out of "paralysands" cries out for Federal Investigation. This was reported in the NY Post, and quickly suppressed.

Likewise, the skewed logistics regarding "co-morbidities" and extreme mortality rate among the elderly.

Yes, I am asking for a serious and intense official inquiry into the likelihood that Senior Citizens were murdered in NY Hospitals, subsequent to the removal of the organs. Why were no official autopsies made? Were the "refrigerated trucks" outside the notorious "Elmhurts" (sic) Hospital just "set dressing?" Plenty of agencies in NYC and Brooklyn, ready, willing and able to supply "location" sets for movie companies. So why not for the Dept of Defense, for example, or the NIH, or CDC or...???

There is no therapeutic justification for the proning of sick persons experiencing respiratory distress.

Perhaps, under the transplanted, wannabe transgender, Dr. Richard aka Rachel Levine, this also occurred in PA. Levine started to transfer elderly patients from hospitals to nursing homes, where they continued to die at a horrendous rate, *but not from infection.*

I have no proof, nor any protected source in this case, but reason *shouts* that the same protocols were in place in PA's Nursing Homes as in NY and PA's Hospitals.

Reason also questions Levine's sudden change of name and gender from Dr. Richard Levine, NY Psychiatrist and Director of a residential home for minors with eating disorders, to Dr Rachel Levine Health Chief of PA, and now, another radical change or "transition" after the PA "Covid" nursing home scandal, to Admiral in a skirt. Perfect for climbing up the rigging...

Confused? Multi-talented? Or something far more sinister, such as avoiding litigation, for injury to, or death of, minors in the residential home for children?

Richard-Rachel certainly did not want his mother to undergo the "Nursing Home" treatment and so he moved her into a hotel.

At the time, three star hotels across the USA were filled with homeless persons and at least one motel in Maryland had a number of AIDs patients.

Not good enough for Mrs. Levine, however !

Paralysands are used in the removal of organs from living patients, a common practice in China, and now, in the USA.

Did Fauci bring this criminal practice from China to the USA? Another exercise in sociopathy?

The patients are alive, aware, given paralysands to prevent movement, but not anaesthesia to block pain. They weep in agony as they are placed face down and their organs are sliced out from the back, the heart, being the last to be removed to keep the others "fresh!" They feel every cut.

At the time of "Covid,"PA's Sec of Health was a man pretending to be a woman. Whether he believes it or is hiding from litigation relevant to previous employment as a psychiatrist working with vulnerable teenagers is relevant to the mental health and motivation of Richard aka Rachel Levine.

Added to that, his experience is primarily in New York City. I have considerable experience with the corruption and evil of NYC and NYS toward the weak, sick and dying. NY's medical officer is Michael Levine.

Richard aka Rachel Levine, the NY shrink with the ongoing identity crisis who controlled PA's Health Services during the "scamdemic" needs to be held accountable. In compromising the health and lives of PA's Seniors, Levine's actions are questionably consistent with those of the dying State of NY, a State executed by its own Governor, Mario Cuomo, now "retired," and Levine's "homeground."

In every action Levine had the full consent and co-operation of then Governor Thomas Wolfe.

Pfizer, GSK, Merck have factories and "research" projects in PA, in Montgomery County an area known for corruption and legal abuses.

Pfizer's factory is visible on the train track to Princeton. GSK is off a quiet street in West Conshohocken, almost hidden from view. Train tracks cross the street from GSK's quarters and disappear into a leafy arbor...and from thence, to anywhere they choose, silently, invisibly, discretely.

Nazi Germany came instantly to mind.

Allegations re the conduct of Pfizer's staff and the treatment of their laboratory test creatures post experiment are extremely disturbing.

-30- April 12, 2022

4. COVID – IN BRIEF   (Dec 2019)

I first encountered "Covid 19"*before it had a name.* In conferring with patients in Europe and the USA, I heard such declarations as: "It's like the flu, but not exactly like the flu. *It's really nasty." "Like flu plus..."*

The most common symptoms were:

- *Fever, low, rarely spiking above 101 – indicating possible depression of the immune system?*
- *Intense weakness, from severe paresis to sensations of complete paralysis.*
- *Utter prostration and exhaustion.*
- *"Heaviness" in limbs.*
- *Complete loss of taste or smell.*
- *Sensitivity to foods, but without consciousness of adverse tastes and odors.*
- *Night sweats – mostly with persons on medications or with vulnerabilities.*
- *"Really nasty" i.e. intense symptoms* lasted a few, intense days, followed by...
- ...a week or two of "feeling not quite "with it"…"like a prolonged hangover that just would not go away…"
- *Restriction-constriction of costal muscles and diaphragm – as if paralysed.*
- *Prolonged loss of taste and smell.*

While most symptoms are consistent with "flu," some symptoms were bizarre, e.g., what appeared to be the "paralysis" of intercostal muscles. What did Fauci or his "sino-entourage" add or allow to be added to the Flu vaccine[8] *of 2019 to elicit such symptoms??? Rodent saliva? Bat spit? Curare? AZT?* Histamine? Mercury? What were the ingredients of his diabolical "cocktail" aka the flu vaccine of 2019!

I treated each patient individually and appropriately according to Homeopathic protocols. Was able to negotiate LOW FLOW Oxygen for the more seriously compromised, i.e., those who came from orthodox medicine with established diagnoses and in a state of panic and terror.

I also strongly recommended back massage – upwards and outwards - or the use of a heated "massage" blanket. NOT the weighted ones, but anything and everything to keep the blood circulating in the vascular system and with it maintain the oxygen intake so vital for the functioning of brain, heart and lungs...indeed, every vital organ and cell in my beloved patients.

For the sequelae, appropriate vitamins and oxygen boosting supports proved extremely helpful and comforting to the patient. Some such oxygen supports are available over the counter in sports outfitters and chain pharmacies

By January I suspected an engineered virus with a *rodent*[9] component, and possible addition of Histamines. As the intel community might put it, there was abundant "chatter" re Fauci's influence on UNC[iv] and collusion with a Chinese

---

[8] April '23. New allegations re snake venom in the "vax" as responsible for clotting. Most snake venoms are haemorrhagic.
[9] Experts claim bats are *not* "rats with wings."

female biochemist, who allegedly brought the contaminated flu vax to Wuhan for mass production.

Patients presented with the usual symptoms of flu...most after taking a flu shot or exposed to "shedders..."

The patients who recovered within 24 hours were exposed to patients with active "influenza" or "vaccinosis," but did not, themselves, receive the vaccine.

Others enjoyed partial recovery, i.e., functional but with residual symptoms. Sadly, the few such patients were so fed up with inertia and delighted to be functional, that they did not follow through to complete the cure.

One unusual symptom appeared in the vaxed flu patients and that was an apparent "paralysis" or paresis of the diaphragm and intercostal muscles. My patients were treated with the appropriate Homeopathic remedy and back massage, always upward and outward, so this symptom, intense, uncomfortable and alarming, seldom lasted more than a few hours, or a day at the most.

It provided the rationale for "venting!"

The patients who received the 2019 flu vaccines usually developed symptoms of intercostal paresis on the second or third day...treated best with the **precise** Homeopathic remedy and /or back massage, upward and outward, or a vibrating "massage" blanket - *unweighted.*

Once that symptom was manifest and treated, the patient recovered rapidly. That seemed to be the critical point...

Flu vaccinated patients would be *referred to me or sought alternative protocols after diagnosis and inability to shake off symptoms produced by the vaccines, ie, "vaccinoses."*

The afore-mentioned unusual symptoms best described as a form of paralysis or paresis of the costal muscles[10] – may have been "engineered" into the 2019 flu vaccine at the UNC laboratories to "justify" the insertion of a vent, and thus provide the "excuse" for tissue rupturing high pressure oxygen. "Rationale" is too dignified a word for that process! That paresis "symptom," or it's precipitant may have been deliberately inserted into the flu vax of 2019 by the Chief of the Ghoul School himself, one Anthony Fauci who must investigated for any possible role in the development of both the 2019 flu vaccine, developed in N. Carolina and brought to Wuhan for mass production and in the so called "anti covid" "vaccine." Mercury is one *possible* culprit. Snake venom is the newest "discovery."

Fauci is the celebrated head of the NIAID...nutty as a squirrel's hide in his constant self-contradictions and ability to talk for hours without saying anything of significance during almost three years of a manufactured health crises and a higher salary than the President of the USA! Not to mention the decades spent corrupting the CDC, NIH, NIAID, FDA, beyond recognition, beyond even the pretence or semblance of *foundational ethics!*

In return for this, he has given a new word to science.

Id est, "SOY-ence," as in fake research, false premises, faked hypotheses, death jabs and confirmation of Stalin's principle, that "if you make a lie big enough, everyone will believe it!"

---

[10] "costals" elevate the ribs on signal from the diaphragm in order to facilitate respiration.

The foul cheat was not working alone. It would be a big mistake to accept him as the lone scapegoat or "useful idiot" – another charming term and praxis deriving from the Soviet era and to allow the intense network of criminal politicians, bureaucrats, dictators, and other megalomaniacal abusers who supported and enabled him to go free. He was the happy "star" of a huge show with a huge "supporting" cast, and powerful, covert, producers...

Fauci has deep connections with Wuhan and China's Xi Jing Ping and Italy's former dictator, Mario Draghi, the co-facilitator of China's colonisation of Northern Italy, i.e. Lombardia, and a possible facilitator of the Dominion election cheating machine. Fauci's name may sound Italian, but to this amateur etymologist it's a combination of "Faux" or "false" and "Ci" for "xi" or...CHINA.

Why are billions of dollars given to such fraudulent and corrupt, self-serving people, when the extraordinary, gentle protocol of authentic Homeopathy can do so much more for a patient than all the punitive measures dreamed up in the sadistic laboratories of Pfizer-GSK, ModeRNA, etc.? *And save billions for the taxpayer!*

Is it because genocide is the new "abortion?

I said it in 1973: the first generation to approve of abortion will be the first to be euthanised and genocided. In 1970 I wrote of the cult of "Thanatos."

Once more, I wish I were wrong...

Homeopaths save lives, *cure* disease and save taxpayers and insurance providers gazillions of dollars while assuring future generations of *healthy populations*.

"Gain of function" research is not for the benefit of humanity. On the contrary, the "gain" desired is not protection but LETHALITY!

Its goal is the creation of **bioweapons** with which to threaten the entire world and mass murder those whom they deem a threat or non-essential to the service of their super luxurious, decadent lifestyles. Mass murder already in process. (2019 and continues through 2023.)

We've already had that "rehearsal" via a self-limiting pseudo virus that "escaped from a Wuhan laboratory..."

WRONG. That was engineered by Fauci and cohorts either in UNC, Chapel Hill and sent to China for mass production or in China itself.[11] It was introduced with the flu "vaccine" of 2019.

That is my contention, and it is based on observation and experience treating flu patients, who had either received the "fauci'd" vax or was in close proximity to vax shedders as well as multiple protected sources.

The timing, the duration, the general and specific symptoms all point to a bio engineered flu vaccine in

---

[11] Reliable but protected sources.

2019 *which did not kill as many as intended and fizzled out in January 2020 or sooner.*

The incubation periods, the prodrome, the sequelae all pointed to a sinister factor, i.e.:

Intent to kill.

But it killed relatively few and those patients not at the mercy of Elmhurst Hospital, NYC and Dr Richard-Rachel Levine of PA recovered rapidly, some with "carryover" syndromes or concommitants due to medications. The mortality rate from flu vax 2019 and

seasonal dispositions was nowhere as high as anticipated and so the iatrogenic murders began.

Murders in hospitals, fake diagnoses, medical equipment, e.g., "ventilators" set at high pressure to puncture lungs, isolation and separation from families, Remdesivir to destroy the kidneys, creating edema (oedema) and softening the lungs for the death jets of highly pressurised oxygen. Where resistance was high, then Midozalam, the "euthanasia" drug finished them off. While their loved ones tried desperately to enter the hospitals to save them, the patient was proned face down and paralysed, tears streaming down their agonised faces, the surgeons carefully carved out their organs, leaving the heart till last, of course, to keep the organs as fresh as possible for sale.

Was there an exceptional need for human transplants at that time, and if so, why?

Back to Euthanasia: Sorry to burst the illusion of a "peaceful, dignified death," but the physical "construction" of the complex and exquisite human anatomy is designed for the preservation and continuation of life.

Take one of those death pills and the body will fight – or want to fight...imagine a mind that decides it didn't like the meds, that it wanted to LIVE after all, but is paralysed, cannot speak, cannot fight, just has to cope with the flood of epinephrenes trying to maintain the heartbeat, to keep the diaphragm pumping, to maintain consciousness while the mind sinks deeper and deeper into the oblivion, and who knows what awaits there..."when we have shuffled off that mortal coil" or "die to sleep, to sleep perchance to dream – but in that sleep of death *what dreams might come...*"[v]

Where natural death occurs a complex process occurs to ease the final moments of a person's earthly existence, but euthanasia starts internalised WARFARE!

We hear so many reports of a smile on the face of the naturally deceased, especially those who die surrounded by family, and who have the privilege of Last Rights.

I hear no such reports of smiles and peace on the faces of those who choose euthanasia. I'm sure that after this statement, mainstream media will oblige with a flood of stories created to justify and promote euthanasia, but the reality is, euthanasia is no longer an explorative search for methodologies to ease the stress of "death throes" in those who are *already exiting* "the mortal coil,[13] and do not have the benefits of the Catholic Sacraments, or other lesser adjuncts that ease suffering and anxiety without promoting or accelerating death.

Euthanasia is now cold blooded, pre-meditated mercenary medical murder.

As I warned in 1972 – the first generation to allow abortion will be the first generation to undergo euthanasia – in its many vicious forms, the latest, of course, being the "covid" "protocols" with the toxic, irreversible, bioweapon falsely presented as a "vaccine."

After all, depopulation is being visited on our children by the "Love, Peace" and Togetherness" generation! Would the "hippies," "stoners," "LSD" cult and commune dwellers want to do us harm?

Yes!

The children of hippy boomers who sang "give peace a chance" are now chanting "Kill babies" and "kill the seniors" "Steal their organs," "Ban the toxic male," etc., and engaging in intensely evil practices including maximising the abortion mortality rate with associate horrors and persuading little children to mutilate their sweet, precious bodies!

We now have generations born to previous generations of psychotropic drug users. It's almost "normalised." *Distressed DNA, ripe for ruinous mRNA!*

---

[13] William Shakespeare, Hamlet's soliloquoy

Psychotropes are flying off the prescription pads of licensed doctors as rapidly as the street dealers sell theirs! Psychotropes were a common factor in the majority of "school shooting."

Daily, the "born addicted" die in the streets of the USA from fentanyl or drugs tainted with fentanyl. Drugs, the ultimate weapons of mass destruction!

Who or what decided to call the Bicentennials "Gen X?" And then designated our wonderful "Zoomers" as Gen Z, ie the *end* of the line, the human species beloved of God finally exterminated. No more offspring of a loving man and woman, husband and wife? Some bizarre "revenge of the nerd" fantasy about creating future generations of "wookies" and ape-men and self-replicating robots? Courtship now is rare, de-personalised "hook-ups" seem to be the standard modus operandus for love-starved, parentally deprived youth.

Even more alarming, childbirth is reduced to an "excremental act" for "transgenders," by the insertion and expulsion of "bum babies," silicon objects, into the rectum.

Transgenderism is the penultimate expression of self-hatred, too often followed by the *ultimate,*[vi] which is suicide.

"Data indicate that 82% of transgender individuals have considered killing themselves and 40% have attempted suicide, with suicidality highest among transgender youth..." https://pubmed.ncbi.nlm.nih.gov/32345113/

And yet, transgenderism is pushed in schools, in media, in "equality" groups, in the offices of compromised social workers, degenerate sociopathic health professionals (not all doctors, obviously) all fully aware of the devastating and **irreversible consequences.**

Hard to find honest recent studies, but in 2016 the Williams Institute (UCLA School of Law)[vii] reported that the percentage of transgender persons identifying as white was **83%**. African American "transgender" stats are dramatically lower.

This is arguably a direct consequence of the abuse and discrimination enacted against white minors in the USA.

So another paragraph in the "Handbook of genocide."

In 1970 I wrote about "Thanatos" or the cult of death, starting with the legalised slaughter of pre-natal infants, the most sadistic, brutal, vile, evil disgusting, irreversible, inexcusable act ever committed by one human against another. In 1973, using testimony known to be false, the Supreme Court of the USA passed the baton of Nazi Germany to their physicians, giving them the "Right" to continue the works of the warped and evil doctors of Hitler's deadly regime.

I have spoken with justices of some of Europe's Supreme Courts, who likewise legitimised abortion.

They were absolutely clueless with regard to the procedures used.

Abortion is *not* an ideological issue. If I were to demonstrate abortion methodology using, say, a teddy bear, and put the video on you tube or facebook, it would be shut down in a nano second and I would be the most vilified person on "planet social media." Abortion is vile.

The long term, cumulative effect of abortion, of the slaughter of 70 million babies – that we know of – is one of collective guilt, universal silence, post abortion syndrome, and, it would seem, that at some level, humanity must feel as if they deserve punishment, and "Covid" was that punishment.

Why else would the general public acquiescently comply with the most appalling, punitive, protocols?

Against medical advice, some patients struggled to work during their "Covid" i.e., vaccinoses out of financial necessity. Again, the lower income patients took the brunt, but survived. Beer, wine, cinnamon!

Future "celebrity guests" of the "Cuckoos' Nest" celebrated their "vaccines," just as they celebrated the in utero butchery of their pre-natal infant, or their castrations and cliterodectomies. – but the **majority of world citizens, the regular workers who keep the world turning, were bullied and blackmailed into taking the "cloth shot"/ pseudo vax, human-bestial genetic modifier.**

After I kicked up in social media, my only outlet at the time, the cabal ceased calling it a "vaccine," and had the effrontery and arrogance to call it "gene **therapy!"**

NOTHING THERAPEUTIC ABOUT IT!

5. FOLLOW THE "SOY-ENCE."

The "virus" aka post 2019 flu vaccinosis appeared to peak in January and start to die off circa late Jan 2020.

The fact that NIH etc., went into overdrive with scare tactics even as it started to decline, leads me to suspect that Fauci and Xi were anticipating far greater damage than that which had already occurred.

Cuomo showed no concern for "Covid" until President Trump mentioned a $2 trillion bail out and a $39k Federal BOUNTY for each CV19 death. Suddenly NYC was the epicenter of the scamdemic, complete with set dressing worthy of a horror movie and what city "set dresses" better than NYC!

"Mortuary" trucks parked outside the City Hospitals – for weeks. *And not a single official autopsy! Seriously?*

Then again, I know for a fact that autopsies in NYC can be rigged so no credibility there, either. Tom Henry has three death certs!

This is significant, as the mortality rate suddenly soared in NY and other bankrupt, Democrat run States. "Death by ingrown toenail *with* Covid!" $13,000 per diagnosis...! $50,000 minimum per corpse! Some MDs, finally finding the courage to protest, estimated the final profit per hospital as 200k per "Covid" patient!

Aside from the relatively innocuous symptomology, the alarm rose to fff (fortissimo) after a news item in the NY Post mentioned that NYC Hospitals were running out of "paralysands."

These are substances like curare or curare compounds that paralyse a conscious patient prior to removing his/her organs against his or her will, a nasty practice developed on China's political prisoners and imported to the USA.

Did Fauci bring this practice to the USA? Is there a desperate need for "donated" organs for transplant? If so, where are American organs sent? Was organ theft the reason for the proning, paralysing and high pressure venting on patients *without* respiratory symptoms, but given fake "with covid" diagnoses?

"Proning" compromised patients was criminal, if not downright cruel and sadistic…

Proning facilitates organ removal from living patients. China uses this method to murder political prisoners, ie, the anti- Communist opposition, while simultaneously profiting from the illicit, criminal, sale of their organs.

Again, in my professional opinion and personal experience with oxygen, **pushing pressured oxygen into damaged lungs is nothing short of murder.**

Damaging lungs through the use of Remdesivir, a "kidney killer," which causes oedema, or fluid build-up in limbs and organs prior to puncturing them with high pressure oxygen is also nothing short of pre-meditated murder. In other words, criminal.

Later, covert autopsies performed in the USA and Italy showed punctures in the lungs of "Covid" patients locked into Hospital rooms and Nursing homes.

I started to sound the alarms on social media, letters to Editors, to the White House and directly to President Trump. Whether my notifications end up in the Presidential Library remains to be seen...but, as with references to my influence in changing the treatment and understanding of AIDs, they are all on public record, somewhere or the other.

I often wonder whether President Trump really had "Covid 19" or if that was a ruse to verify my allegations for himself.

He set up a massive Covid Emergency Center in the Javits Center in NY and brought in a massive Hospital ship.

No one came, revealing that the mass induced hysteria was for nought, but cui bono – why? Land and asset grab from the "Boomers?" Proliferation of 5Gs? Other covert activity?

The venting stopped. The Nursing Home deaths were exposed. **People stopped dying and started to recover.**

Trump called their bluff – and paid a price for it.

The masks came off – in more ways than one - and continue to be removed, now that the CDC and taxpayer funded, profiteering, pHARMaceutical "giants" are increasingly obliged to submit information

and data to Congress, Courts, Public Agencies and grieving families.[viii]

In brief, so called "COVID" ie, flu plus, is nasty, but seldom fatal, even for the elderly, until and unless they are bullied into hospital admission on any excuse, paltry, false, sometimes valid but irrelevantand thence to a painful, lonely, agonising, death by pulmonary puncture or organ theft.

Whatever the sinister reason for creating two years of terror and house arrest, the truth is that people were put to death. Citizens of a Republic were murdered. In cold blood.

Even with the rapid closure of the Covid Emergency Center and the Hospital Ship due to **'no takers," ie no epidemic /scamdemic / plandemic / shamdemic,** the general public was still sufficiently terrified into taking the newest "headliner," the CLOTSHOT, the deathjab, the "covid "vaccine" i.e. genocidal bioweapon!

Now that the general populations have been convinced to take the gene destroying bioweapon aka "vaccine," a genuine pandemic is in full swing. However, it is not "contagious" per se; it is *"transmitted" from doctor to patient* via a **syringe** *filled with the RNA of monkeys, rats,* aborted baby tissue and Heaven knows what else.

Snake/ophidian venom is usually haemorrhagic, ie, caused prolonged bleeding, but some are thrombotic.

Bats and snakes[14] are "contenders," but no confirmation, either from source, nor officialdom, as yet.

Am I the only scientist in the world who saw the lethality of the "clotshot" on first reading the initial ingredients?

Was it my training in and studies of the human immune system via the exquisite Science of Homeopathy that alarmed me to an excruciating degree when the presence of simian and rodent RNA in those "vaxes" was revealed. Homeopathy is vastly superior. Even so, it's hard to believe that the "old school" of pharma medicine is that daft!

Fauci had to know. The FDA, NIH, NIAID, CDC, DOD, WEF, WHO, selected Heads of State et al – all knew! It was **state sponsored pharma terrorism!**

Fauci "officially" retired in December 2022, but is still working ex officio, burying the "bodies" no doubt.

More suspicious "accidental" fires no doubt!

Follow the "soy-ence," and **PROSECUTE FAUCI NOW!**

---

[14] April 2023 - Snakes are now suspected contenders for the clotting factor in the death jabs. Snake venom is usually haemorrhagic!

6. "SCAMDEMIC" OR "CLINICAL TRIAL" OF BIOWEAPON AKA COVID VACCINE.

As night follows day, flu season follows flu vax season!

Flu vaccinations preceded the 1918 flu epidemic which targeted a vulnerable, grieving malnourished population post WWI and murdered them.

In that and other 20th century epidemics, patients of **Homeopaths** enjoyed a 94-96% full recovery rate, despite the "dumping" of **pharm**a's very sick patients on our hospitals.

I refer to ***authentic* Homeopaths**, not the HYBRIDS promoted these days by the compromised "alphabet" agencies, working for the **pharm**aceutical industry instead of the public whom they are *mandated to protect*! The alliance between Deep State and Big Pharma is incestuous and its product is consequently deficient.

I have *potential* solutions to the sudden deaths of athletes in particular, but with the mRNA factor this is a challenge, even for an authentic, experienced, Homeopath. Potentials but no test facility.

Just as I provided solutions in the AIDS epidemic at a Dept of State conference.[15] This cost Fauci and the AZT

---

[15] Circa 1983 – I had no official status then so I provided answers in the form of questions. Understand and treat of AIDs changed drastically.

pushers dearly. The anagram's true meaning? *Acquired Immune Deficiency from XS use of antibiotics!*

While I am sick and tired of "giving away" my "Nobels," that is, knowledge and insights acquired the hard way and unique to me, the suffering of humanity has accelerated, thanks to Fauci, Xi Jing, Draghi, Obama, Biden, and other promoters of the Nazi driven pharmaceutical industry. It has now reached a point where I am conscience bound to speak up regardless of the plagiarists.

"Fools, let them take it...for there's more enterprise in walking naked!" W.B.Yeats

Bayer, Pfizer, EU, WEF, Schwab, Soros, Von Leyen, etc., all have strong, irrefutable roots and lines going back to Hitler's Gestapo. Sad to say the Bush/Scherf family also have historical "credits" for supplying the Third Reich with necessities and equipment from the USA, grossly violating the law, but protected from consequences.

The "scamdemic" proved that the CDC is not a competent authority when it comes to the health and safety of the citizens of the United States of America.

But is it even honest! Or just, hopelessly, inept.

There are abundant links to the CDC's vacillations and collusion with the Pharmaceutical industry that it is mandated to monitor. See end of book.

THE **toxicity of the "vaccines"** aka Clot shots, aka death jabs, aka any number of pseudonyms necessary to discuss the subject on social media, should have been as **perfectly**

obvious to any half way competent biochemist, physician, pharmacist *as it was to me, immediately, instantly, without hesitation when I first read the contents of the vial!*

I knew this would be the hardest challenge to even the finest authentic Homeopath! It's not like antidoting snake poison, for example.

How and why did NIH et al allow ModeRNA, with its simian RNA, and Pfizer with canine kidney tissue, aborted baby tissue, alleged HIV RNA, and Johnson now J and J, with what appears to be RODENT RNA...to inject these lethal almost irreversible substances into a baby's arm, a senior's arm, an adult arm, any arm...without question or protest. And now the bragging "I got my shot" celebrities are dying off. So tragically.

Did anyone ever question the wisdom or authenticity of testing drugs on animals, on prisoners, on drug addicts or persons with immune and other systems previously damaged or even wrecked during previous "clinical trials?"

And did the CDC allow Fauci and UNC's doctored 2019 flu' shot to be mass produced in Wuhan and then brought back to the USA? If so, – how and what was the motivation of the CDC in not only allowing, but in aiding and abetting the iatrogenic murder and/or manslaughter of millions of Americans?

Speaking of murder – when will the media speak the truth about the hospital and nursing home deaths of "vaccinated" patients...poisoned, proned, (squishing the diaphragm is such a good idea (sarcasm) for patients with respiratory issues) and then subjected to pressurised oxygen, bursting into and through their sodden "wet sponge" lungs...

WHAT KIND OF PEOPLE ARE THEY??? Carryovers from Nazi Germany? Because they definitely merit a Nuremberg trial, along with Fauci, Gates, Bourla, von Leyen, and the European Governments that took their lead from the CDC and NIH and also killed their own people.

Then again, with Ursula von Leyen, daughter of Hitler's senior SS Officer, Herr Ernst Albrecht, as President of the "European Union," and wife of a Pfizer chief executive and bioweapons, erratum, "vaccine" salesman, and WWII collaborators, ie, West Ukraine, slurping up billions in "Aid" money, for ulterior purposes, the "deep state." the Karl Schwabs, the disappearing – but not declared dead - public figures, the world is starting to look and feel a lot like a FOURTH REICH!

For my attempts to protect the American people, I lost my home, and survived two attempts on my life, the latter after proving the superiority of *authentic* Homeopathy in the treatment of MRSA, thrombosis, paralysis, etc., in hospital. So I know already how compromised the **pharma** – medical cartels can *be*.

And shockingly, the extents to which they will go to destroy even one, very excellent, *authentic* Homeopath.

Attempted murder, August 2006 and Nov 2, 2006 was my "reward" for saving the State of New York *millions* while substantially improving the life and health of long term patients. This after my research proposal past six committees and then probably landed on Fauci's desk.

"Vaccines," ALL OF THEM, are iatrogenic, that is, damaging and destructive to our very genomes, our mitochondrial DNA - the very structure and balance of our unique and irreplaceable bodies, "knit in our mothers' wombs..." Psalm 139

The mRNA bioweapons are the most dangerous of them all.

They destroy our very essence. Once the bestial RNA burrows into our blood, bones, sinews, brains, we are no longer fully human. We have allowed ourselves to become genetically modified hybrids – humanoid rodents, monkey-men, planet of the Apes, etc.,etc. However, that bestial RNA is rejected by mature immune systems, all too often only after clots start to form and mitochondrial proteins initiate a teratogenic formation.

These formations are ultimately rejected but their presence in the body obstructs blood flow and alarms the immune system into aggressive "attack mode,"e.g., fevers, elevated heart and respiration rates, etc.

A pre-natal baby's immune system is immature and their cellular intelligence cannot recognise or defend against the cerebral brain cells of other creatures.

Why do Pfizer scientists take the brain cells of living prenatal human infants – acquired from abortuaries – and implant them in the brains of very young rodents?

Who funds those vile experiments and for what purpose?

I have observed the results of some of these more intense hybridising experiments in dark labs in Europe, possibly

Ukraine. They are beyond imaginable evil, images one would never wish to witness or carry in ones traumatised memory.

In these vile cases, embryonic cells were used.

The attempts to GMO adults are a mega disaster from the POV of the p-harm-a industry and their Fauci ghouls. No doubt they have taken notes and will try again.

But meanwhile, millions are dying, daily, from an experiment in the mass-modification of the human species. Transhumanism in every imaginary form.

Did they learn nothing from the use of equine oestrogen as "replacement" hormone therapy for humans? That therapy has since fallen into disfavor due to the high incidence of mammary and uterine cancers following such treatments. But, (sarcasm) *nil desperandum,* the trillion dollar **pharm**a industry is researching away - at the taxpayers' expense, and is sure to come up with a product that is even more deadly.

That is the meaning of Generation Z. The last fully human Generation.

If Schwab et pals have their way, the majority of humans will be genetically modified minions, "wookies," under the control of R2D2, etc.

Mega investor in transhuman robots... Jeffrey Epstein...!

I wrote "Homeopathy in the Time of Covid," in 2022, self-published, but I do not trust the CDC, NIH, etc., to respect its integrity. You may buy a bunch of copies and learn something.

For the record, "Tick borne disease" also responds exquisitely to *authentic* Homeopathic treatment in my experience.

For the record, if Covid were a genuine pandemic, CDC and NIH etc., would receive a giant "F" (Fail) for the absurd protocols put in place to "protect" us... I've seen toddlers show more concern and intelligence in the care of their sick siblings or parents than the dancing ghouls of America's hospitals!

Similarly the absurdity of coercive masking!

If they want my advice, they can **pay me twice Fauci's salary!**

What were the CDC, NIH, NIAID, and the rest of the "alfalfabet" gang thinking?

Were they thinking? Or "calculating?" Or "colluding" in depopulation agendae?

Or were they just counting the "bean bags?"

The CDC has greatly harmed the USA, and by extension, the world.

The CDC Senior Boardroom Officers must resign immediately and these absurd, bigoted "enquiries" cease and desist.

After all, if they can condone the products used to torture little babies to death in utero, they have already hit the lowest of the low. Add to that the sale of organs carved out of living, suffering babies, whose vocal cords are cut in order to silence their agonised cries. What have we become, Lord, what have we become!

If the "alfalfabets" and p-harm-a can allow the Boston college bio weapons labs to produce GENOCIDAL BIO WEAPONS, and possibly even fund them, then they are building a dungeon for themselves of murder and iatrogenic violence, out of which they may never climb. Bratislava's Museum of Torture comes to mind!

I recommend that they cease and desist from pushing vials of toxic, "unmetabolisable" substances on infants and children with fragile immune systems and seniors – who, by definition, have sturdy immune systems; likewise the military, and leave our sturdy workers and parents to live in peace and **good health**. CDC and p-harm-a execs are free to indulge in as many clot shots as they choose for themselves, as long as they keep their *shedding* far from the aforesaid public.

Interestingly, p-harm-a's "health execs," corporate execs, politicians, diplomats and media were all exempt from the gross, unjust and destructive travel restrictions between the USA and Europe and "mandatory" jabs![16]

It is also likely that these exemptions were global.

"Lords and Serfs" do not belong in a Republic.[ix]

Especially a Republic whose people fought so hard and suffered so much to bring "Liberty and Justice" to all...and by extension, serves as a "shining city on a hill" to the world at large.

Move them out!

[1616] Latest walk back as of late April 2023 is that the "vaccines" did not contain mRNA. I know my keyboard is ghosted of late, possible spyware in place.

Or more effectively, perhaps, call in the **exorcists!**

7. NATURAL IMMUNITY vs "VACCINATION"

Vaccines are the "devil's walking parody"[17] of the human immune system and Homeopathy.

Vaccines besiege, bombard, confuse and overwhelm the human immune system at the best of times. Bad enough when "one size fits all, but when mixed with other pathogens, bestial mitorobosomes, mRNA, ATPs, etc., they inevitably become *lethal.* The human immune system, brilliant and complex *qua meme,* is not designed to absorb, identify and fight the deadly "cocktails" allegedly produced by Ukraine and China's secret laboratories, financed and driven by the USA, be it Fauci's NIH, Biden, Obama, Xi Ping, etc.,

Then there's the newly revealed involvement of the US Depart of Defense.[18]

At the very beginning, circa 1796, Jenner's[19] cowpox-smallpox vaccine killed his own son and many of his neighbours. He was about to give up when the p*harm*aceutical industry took over.   There was *one*

---

[17] G.K. Chesterton "The Donkey"

[18] https://www.defense.gov/Spotlights/Coronavirus-DOD-Response/Latest-DOD-Guidance/https://www.army.mil/article/264274/army_rescinds_covid_19_vaccination_requirements
https://www.defense.gov/News/Releases/Release/Article/2310994/us-government-engages-pfizer-to-produce-millions-of-doses-of-covid-19-vaccine/

[19] Edward Jenner invented the cowpox-smallpox vaccine circa 1794.

pathogen in his shot, *one only, and yet it proved lethal to his son and heir and half his village!*

This is not mentioned in his "Wiki" biography. While they display a photo of an Italian statue of Jenner injecting, thereby killing, his naked son, with cowpox "venom," they make no mention of that salient fact.

The vaccines – vacco = cow - cowpox vs smallpox appears to be "inspired" by Homeopathy, but is actually ISOPATHIC rather than Homeopathic. Homeopathy gently stimulates and with *precise remedy selection* by an expert Homeopath, *coaxes* the immune system to life, elevates the opsonic indices, gently, stage by stage in order to protect the vulnerable energies of the suffering patient.

We do *not* replace one set of *allopathics* or *antagonists* with another.

Chemicals and pharmaceuticals have been developed *in vitro, ie* in sterile glass vials under controlled, uniform conditions, and stabilised temperatures.

They are then tested on "isometric" lab rodents. Their systems bear little similarity to the complexities of the human biome. Samples are then imposed on "professional" testers whose immune systems are already damaged by years of "prostitution" to the p-*harm*-a industries.

These are sometimes students or prisoners, trying to earn *ex officio* "time credits" and money for their families. They may be drug addicts with cross addictions. They maybe already on multiple meds, and if low income students, very likely on a minimalist, low nutrition, diet.

Result = RESULT COMPROMISED!!!

Testing for ModeRNA killed an estimated 476 human "guinea pigs" in the first *months* of "clinical trials,' and still was pushed onto the market, where it continues its deadly work and has been banned by the FDA along with its cohort Pfizer!

In Montana, steps are being taken by their legislature to criminalise the use of "vaccinated" blood in transfusion.

The official CDC site [20] also reveals a mountain of similarly disturbing statistics.

Newsweek:[21] "There are hundreds of reports of people having died after getting a COVID vaccine, but that *"does not necessarily mean*" the vaccine was the cause," and...

Sure!

"Our VAERS result showed 970 people died after being given a Pfizer or Moderna vaccine shot. Of those deaths, 495 occurred following a Moderna shot, and 475 deaths followed a Pfizer shot. Newsweek contacted Pfizer and Moderna for comment."

Epoch Times first published this information. If Newsweek was attempting "push back" against that information, then Newsweek failed miserably.

---

[20] https://www.cdc.gov/coronavirus/2019-ncov/vaccines/safety/adverse-events.html

[21] https://www.newsweek.com/covid-vaccine-deaths-cause-pfizer-moderna-fact-check-966-died-1574447

Then again, the "deep state creds[22]" of the main stream media are "impeccable" - to the inverse degree that their articles are "credible!"

---

[22] Founded by Time Foreign Ed John Martyn, funded by Mellon, Cheney and John Hay Whitney. Taitsie Mellon married a JH Whitney senior Exec who was later appointed as a US Ambassador by Pres GHW Bush and President George W Bush. (Jnr) Both emerged following intense media criticism of Rothschild involvement in World War I. <Rense.com>

8. About MITOCHONDRIA - mRNA

<u>Mitochondria</u> – energy producing "entities within our cells. "protein producing" proteins manufacturing ATP[23] within cells, *and ... "*[xi].e., organelles (micro organs) in animal and plant cells in which *oxydative phosphylation* takes place.[24]"

Specialised ribosomes within mitochondria help manufacture those proteins. Some maintain or produce Bacteria.

<u>Ribosomes:</u>

i. Tiny protein producing factories with cells, ubiquitous and apparently isometric.

ii. Ribosomes maintaining, i.e., producing *Bacteria are structurally similar to human protein producing ribosomes.*

iii. "Mito-robosome" a protein active in mitochondria, identifies and encodes mRNA into the host DNA.

In other words there are a number of ribosomes: those which produce protein, those which produce bacteria and those that "translate" mitochondrial RNA (mRNA) and knit it into the mitochondrial DNA...

Mitochondrial ribosome or mitoribosome is a protein complex active in mitochondria and functions as a riboprotein for translating mRNA encoded in mitochondrial DNA...

---

[23] Adenosine triphosphate

[24] I note that no two images for mitochondrial-ATP synthesis are alike and that no two definitions of mitochondria are closely alike; while not necessarily contradictory, they do give rise to speculation.

Here's where it gets interesting. *Mitorobosome is attached to inner mitochondrial membrane...where it functions as a riboprotein for "translating" mRNA encoded in mitochondrial DNA.*

Did the Covid "clot shot" trigger a bio crisis whereby the mitochondrial ribosome /mitoribosome "refused" to "translate" mRNA and encode it to or from Mt DNA, i.e., Mitochondrial DNA? Did it start out in "good faith" but then recognise the anomolous RNA and say, "no way, monkey/ rodent/ canine RNA!?" Did it produce the "spike" or APP protein to deter the "recombinants" from recombining?

Did the incomplete hybrid protein / cartilege / tissue then adhere to the inner mitochondrial robosome or attach and remain attached to a vascular or arterial wall and "hang on" till athletic exertion elevated blood pressure, triggering excess heat, etc., which then eroded the adherent fibres freeing the hybrid tissue to go directly to the heart of the victim, causing instant death.

Or again, did it block circulation sufficiently to pool the blood and create thromboses or clots, which then bypassed the teratogenic "obstacle," again going directly to the heart or brain causing instant death?

It appears that the mRNA can be destroyed if the means and methods that I suggested are followed immediately.

To recap: alcohol, as in hot whiskey and soda; if alcohol is contra-indicated, then tonic water, cinnamon, cider vinegar-water-honey, Vits D and E and other anti-coagulants should be taken ASAP, then, daily.

Once the DNA translates genetic information to the mRNA and the mRNA which then transcribes it *-qua "codon"* – into a *protein,* ie, solid new tissue, "knitting" together host DNA and alien mRNA, colloquially speaking, that is, solutions are not so readily available.

Therefore it is imperative to **block the formation and attachment of alien ribosomes, *ab initio.***

None of those functions can occur in the absence of oxygen. However, "oxygen" deprivation is *not* an option. It is possible, that smokers have an advantage...along with persons who enjoy wine with dinner, cinnamon, turmeric, and take Vitamins A , D and E on a regular basis.

It's not as "elemental" as antidoting poison... Poisons can erode and destroy tissue, enzymes, mitochondria, organs and organelles, if allowed, but the accursed mRNA "covid codons" are embedded in or attached to your membranes, cells and tissues, until you find a means of "solution-/absorption elimination," surgery or drop dead from the release of the clot or alien "cartilege" aka "white clots" due to intense activity, raising the body temperature and increasing the blood pressure.

Otherwise healthy activities have become inimical, dangerous.

These cannot be antidoted by medicine. It is a challenge even to precise, Homeopathic means and methodology.

These must be removed by a skilled vascular surgeon; or by a skilled Homeopath.

Now vascular surgeons have already removed these teratogens from the veins and arteries of living "clotshot" victims, just as the funeral directors of England did for the dead, revealing all.

Few survivor/victims have considered consulting professional Homeopaths despite the falsehoods promulgated by pharma meds and the fact that everything viable or helpful in "modern" ie retro medicine has been purloined from the Homeopaths, but without any genuine understand and respect for this extraordinary "art" and science! "Hardest to learn and practice – but the most effective!" John Diamond, MD

Rabbit hole or labyrinth. You decide.

mRNA-1273-P301-Protocol.pdf

More interpretations of Mitochondria. In the world of genetics, no two definitions are identical – fair enough, but one would expect greater or stronger syntheses among true scientists.

For example, Encyclopedia Brittanica describes Mitochondria as *"organelles, (mini organs) in animal and plant cells in which oxydative phosphorylations takes place, ie, minute factories requiring oxygen to generate adenine tri-phosphate (ATP) or release of "usable" energy through chemiosmosis and electron transport chains.*

Retro: Science class, basement of convent high school. Don't they know flames rise upward...oh well, Faith can bring fire engines... Teenage girls in floppy, figure concealing uniforms in "scintillating" heavy grey, school tie mandatory, sit on stools in the tiny science lab while a minute 83 year old nun in classic religious attire, i.e., swathed in flammable cotton, takes a glass vial from the locked cabinet and with tongs, removes a tiny amount of phosphorus from its oily prison smiling as it combusts spontaneously in the presence of oxygen/room air. She replaces the cap on the bottle, replaces it in the cupboard and asks:

"Now, girls, what did you learn...?"

"Not to put science labs in basements of buildings containing hundreds of young students," I respond silently, back aching from the bar stool and the refusal of smug Irish GPs to respect the correct self-diagnosis of an 11 year old and treat accordingly...

9. MITOCHONDRIA

As anticipated from the beginning of the "COVID" charade, it is the interfacing of hostile, alien, bestial mitochondria with the Amyloid Precursor Proteins, colloquially referred to as "Spike proteins" that grab onto the invading RNA causing the anomalous, fibrous adhesions incorrectly described as "clots."

Teratogenic fibrinogens is my term for them, as most anomalies appear not to be blood clots *per se* but malformed proteins produced by the insane attempts of Fauci, Schwab, Gates et al to irreparably damage the purity of the human genome and create trans-species sub humans, eg "wookies," or humanoid robots, eg R2D2 etc., and such as may be found in, say, "Star Wars" – a precursor of "WEF's" covert agendae?

Currently the term "spike protein" has been invented to scare us, when, in fact, they appear to be the "good guys" in this scenario as they *prevent* the rodent RNA and the macaque monkey RNA from combining and er "mating with" the human DNA.

Hybridisation appears to be the goal. Once you are a "re-invented" *patented* subspecies, self-evident **"Inaliable Rights"** no longer apply to you.

Since the content of the junk killer vax is the property of Pfizer, ModeRNA, Janssen (J and J) they are quite capable of convincing their corrupt DC cohorts – with

the usual "currency" incentives – that the post vax dual species is now their property too, and so requisition the poor victim for experimentation.

However, the RNA-DNA splicing appears to have failed.

Either the adhesions kill the victims directly, by blocking blood flow to the heart, or it has created peculiar, "deformed" fibrinogens...inert, non-viable proteinacious tissue that the body rejects, which cling to arterial walls until elevated blood pressure, increased body temperature and accelerated blood flow release into the blood stream, and thence, directly into the vena cava, or deeper into the heart, if small enough, where it blocks the circulation and the patient dies.

These adhesions are increasingly being surgically removed from veins and arteries without killing the victim. This, in part is due to the amazing work of English and American morticians who exposed these anomalies to the world, while the AMA and the Coroner's offices were resoundingly SILENT.

Homeopaths have been repairing genetic anomalies for over two centuries now, but in a manner so exquisite, so refined, so subtle and benevolent that the pHARMa schools can only grind their teeth in frustration and spend millions of dollars to discredit us and advance their own, primitive, systems.

In this process, and with this attitude, they have discarded the better products, used by allopaths and herbalists for centuries.

We were warned: Planet of the Apes, Island of Dr. Moreau, Star Wars, and all the bizarre creatures played by children on unmonitored tablets, phones, computers. Hollywood's "psy ops" are deliberately too far-fetched to be taken seriously by healthy minds.

"SARS-COV is a *synthetic spike protein (APP) chimera (shadow) engineered to attach to human ACE2 receptors and inserted into a recombinant SARSr-COV base.*

(Sounds "off" to me.)

It is more likely a live "vaccine," not yet engineered to a more attenuated, ie developed, virulent, "stable" state that the program sought to create at its final session.

However, it leaked and spread rapidly because it was "aerosolized" so WUHAN could efficiently inject bats in caves, (in order to take the "virus" and attenuate it again??? Otherwise, why*) but "it was not yet ready to infect bats yet, which is why it does not appear to affect bats"*wins the Fauci "peak of inanity" award!"

Are they expecting a cable: "Ready to infect bats. Please advise re time and place. Roger and out."

Seriously! I don't have the sources for that, swamped as I am at present, but it is from one of the official agencies.

I am "swamped" because in late 2022 to early 2023, "mountains" of data became available. Data incompatible with humanity! Data justifying my concerns!

"The reason the "disease" is so confusing is because it is less a virus than an engineered spike protein "hitch-hiking" a ride on a SARS-COVID quasi species swarm... "

The "soyentists" love their colloquialisms, makes them feel less nerdy, God help us! Seriously – "spike protein hitch-hiking a ride on a SARS-COVID quasi species swarm..."????! *Hitch-hiking? Quasi species? Swarm?*

That has to be Fauci – he gets the "Nobel" for the most bizarre mangling and abuse of the English language at the best of times, but "hitch-hiking spike proteins"gets the garbled science award! May this obscene verbiage will "hitch hike" a "ride" into the ethers of oblivion when Fauci faces his final judgment!

"The closer it gets to the final live attenuated vaccine form, the more likely it is that it has been de-attenuating since its initial escape in August 2019."

Talking out of both sides of the mouth perhaps? As it continues to attenuate it's simultaneously de-attenuating? I find the "initial escape" in **August 2019** interesting and wish I had the original source of this fascinating piece.

I have contended from the beginning that the "covid 19" influenza aka "corona virus complete with photo-shopped drier ball" was insinuated into the world via the flu vaccination of 2019. So did the "virus" escape, or was it shipped to the USA under false pretenses?

Either way, a serious crime was committed. And where was the FBI on this? "Hitchiking on a swarm?"

Life Site News publishes excellent articles, the titles of which I shall post here, rather than at the end of the book: However, I reached my conclusions long before I read the following. They were sent by a patient who died because she could not reach me. Due to political harassment I had to leave the USA and become a nomad. These files remained unopened until recently.

The titles, themselves are revealing, and from December 2020!!! *And still they didn't listen.*

8/28/20 by Ethan Huff: "THERE'S ALMOST NO CHANCE A VACCINE FOR COVID-19 WILL WORK AT ALL, WARNS SCIENTIST."

The scientist is Professore Giuseppe Tritto, President of the World academy of Biomedical Sciences and Technology. (WABT)

12/09/20 "DOCTOR ON CNN: DON'T BE "ALARMED" IF ELDERLY DIE AFTER RECEIVING COVID VACCINE..." CDC Panel voted 13:1 to experiment first on elderly staff (?) in long term facilities.

What planet is that man living on: Planet sociopath? Overcrowded with Fauci's associates, the CDC, FDA, NIH, NIAID. The AMA? All of the above are filled with "fear and loathing" of the genius of Homeopathy.

12/21/20 13 PEOPLE DIED DURING MODERNA'S COVID VACCINE TRIAL – Myocarditis, thrombocytopenia, acute kidney failure, obstructive nephrolithiasis, complications, organ failure, then suicide.

That was just ONE patient. Others – facial paralysis, Bells Palsy, "head trauma, "found dead," "uncertain cause" "cardiac arrest," "systemic inflammatory response syndrome in the setting of known malignancy????"

"Known malignancy" and they are still injected with that junk?

And the FDA gave the "go ahead" for further research?

Criminal! Medical terrorism! Aiding and abetting?

12/24/20 "Vaccine COVID = IRREVERSIBLE GENETIC DAMAGE – A CRIME AGAINST HUMANITY."

"THE COVID 19 VACCINE IS AN ACT OF WAR DESIGNED TO CONTROL POPULATION AND GENETICALLY MODIFY HUMANS."

Gratitude to the late, great, Mary Brown of Queens, NY and Mayo, ROI for the foregoing.

Rest in Peace, Mary. I know you are with the angels, your beloved pets and the babies you tried to save outside New York's Hellish abortuaries. You are remembered and forever loved.

10. A "ROSE" IS A ROSE. A BIOWEAPON IS A BIOWEAPON!

One of my early posts on social media.
The "vaccine" is *not* a vaccine.

It was obvious from just reading the contents that this would be a horrendous weapon against humanity.

I might not have used the term "weapon" originally, but it was certainly intended to be lethal.

So much information is now flooding into the "omniverse" to justify my concerns, based on science and logic.

The "clots" are not the problem.

The mRNA is the problem

The "clots" are the **result** of the body trying to take the alien tissue and flow it out of the body.

The alien tissue adheres to the human tissue (dNA ribosomes) by means of mitochondrial messenger, ie bestial mRNA. This invades and interfaces with the human DNA - so that when the immune system's "seek and destroy" cells, T4 and T8" recognise it and trigger the body's defenses to try to push it out, by elevated temperature and increased blood flow, they do not have sufficient force to flush out the fibrins... The circulation is blocked and the blood pools, stagnates and clots within a few minutes – or at the outside, 7-10. This clot may partially or completely block the circulation, and so the heart starves of fluid and cyclo-oxygenase and the patient dies of heart failure, aka myocarditis.

If the RNA-created fibrin fills the veins and blocks the return of blood to the heart, so the heart starves, and, deprived of oxygen, dies, along with the patient. Prothrombin is produced and *the pooled blood clots*.

When the fibrinogen/teratogen partially blocks the blood flow, slowing it down, the blood partially coagulates. The blood either stops flowing or he clots reach the heart, blocking the valves and killing the patient instantly.

When the teratogenic fibrins adhere to the walls of the arteries, allowing some function, this can give time for treatment for the moderately active, but athletes become particularly vulnerable.

An athlete is fit, works to max, increasing blood pressure and accelerating flow. Escalated during competition. The intense heat and pressure then forces "adherent" fibrins off the vascular walls and into the blood stream, thence to the heart, thereby causing the sudden death of the athlete.

Depending on the RNA - and there are several sources in use: macaque monkey, rodent, even poor little prenatal babies, the development of the combo human-bestial fibrins may vary. Latest suspect is the snake.

Some variants may take longer to clog the human vascular system, and or be removed, but it is extremely difficult to consider a safe way to stop them re-growing once the alien RNA is in the system.

Recombinant! Just keeps on combining and recombining, that is, invading your personal territory, ie, DNA until the invading RNA turns you into a hybrid and the real you ceases to exist.

You are trapped inside a stranger's body. Mostly human, but part beast... Where prenatal infants were used the result is the stuff of nightmares. Yes, the secret laboratories of China and East Europe – perhaps the very ones precision bombed by Vladimir Putin.

That's a rather extreme statement, but the conduct and behaviors that I have witnessed in the recently vaxxed upholds it. This includes rodent type behavior, baboon type behavior, aggression, violence, and more in people that I once knew as gentle, normal, sane.

Perhaps even a reflection of the exterior political scenario where communities and nations are invaded by hostile "aliens," their natural habitats destroyed, their freedoms revoked and their identities undermined or eviscerated!

And so they revert to atavism.[25]

---

[25] "The Sanity of Christ vs the Fallacies of Freud" by Dr. D McNamara
"Totem and Taboo" by Sigmund Freud cribbed off RC missionaries.

11. POTENTIAL SOLUTIONS?

Any Homeopathic suggestions would be distorted by the **pharma** shills, so I tread carefully with non Homeopathic professionals, including MDs.

However, there are one or two non-Homeopathic protocols with potential for success in this disastrous area, which I would personally try, if assaulted by one of those toxic needles.

These are neither prescription, nor advice, but are shared *pro bono publico*.

If forcibly poisoned with the human-bestial "GMO" bioweapon fraudulently called a "vaccine" I would *immediately* take a hot whiskey with cloves and cinnamon or any form of alcohol *and anti-coagulants immediately* available, i.e., cinnamon, aspirin, etc.

The heat and alcohol have the potential to erode and break the molecular shell of the alien RNA, which, in its raw state starts to degrade at a temperature of 7F.
Hence the initial shipments of the "covid vaccines" in coolers and refrigerated containers.

Abundant revelations by survivors of "covid jabs" amount to substantial circumstantial evidence in favor of anti-coagulants. I have no proof that this is actually therapeutic in this situation, but it is highly logical.

Survivors of the "clot shot,"aka "deathjab," "gene therapy" "covid vaccine" either regularly used one of the following or a combination or took one of the adjuvants listed below:

Wine, Whiskey, Beer.
Cinnamon,
Turmeric, "turmeric tea..."
Dandelion tea
Aspirin
Cider Vineg
ar in water, w honey and cinnamon
Honey,
Ivermectin
Hydroxychloroquinine/ H2OCLQ sulphate
TONIC WATER (Hydroxyquinine) H2OQ
Prescribed Heparin.
Vitamins A, D,E
Vitamin B12
Kelp

ALL OF THE ABOVE ARE ANTI-COAGULANTS!
ALL OF THE ABOVE PREVENT CLOTTING.

If the "Covid vaccine" were simply a poison, even a laboratory concocted toxin, I could use Homeopathic methods to antidote and eliminate rapidly from system. This worked with:
Attempted arsenic poisoning
Eschar from natural, not weaponised, anthrax
Nicotine poisoning
But "recombinant Messenger RNA" does not work through the digestive or transcutaneous absorption, but directly

through our core mitochondria and DNA. It's a "Kling-on!"

MRNA attacks through the very core and essence of our being: our DNA, our blood, and alters our "zoological" status forever! Like the large African cuckoo which plants its egg in the nest of small birds...and when it hatches exhausts the host birds with its insatiable demands for food. The host's own fledglings die of starvation, and the young cuckoo then flies away.

Pfizer-ModeRNA – JAJ – Astra Z are worse than "cuckoos."

They pervert the natural order by "mating" human DNA with the cruddy mRNA of **another species!**

Imagine the product of mating a cuckoo with a tiny robin or wee wren...nausea inducing. Even if such offspring were to survive – it would have no hope of reproducing.

Horse and donkey can make a mule, but *a mule cannot make another mule!!!*

IS THAT WHY OUR YOUNGSTERS ARE DESIGNATED "GENERATION Z?" THE LAST OF THE LINE?

Is that the plan all along? Throw in abortion, gender bending, transhumanism, the inevitable elevated rate of suicide, nutritional toxicity, etc., and a very few "families" will inherit a mountain of corpses, abandoned buildings, torrid, polluted water and contaminated land.

*Some it will kill; others it will alter, and I have witnessed
aggressive, even animalistic behavior in post "vax"
persons formerly known to be kind and courteous. These
were most often ModeRNA users. Some were mixed, but
the ModeRNA was 99% persistent or consistent in all the
aggressors who behaved like a "pack of baboons." In fact I
suspected simian RNA before the macaque monkey element
was "accidentally" exposed.*

Back to solutions: Those who cannot drink alcohol may
benefit by drinking hot lemonade with cinnamon, honey,
cloves. Or tea with the above, if lemon or cider vinegar is
too acidic.

I would follow with a daily glass of wine – organic
preferably, as sulphates are used to preserve RNA as
well as wine.

This only as a preventative, immediately after the shot.
While "thinner" blood is less likely to force-release
adherents, if taken once the clot or fibrin has formed and is
adhering to a vascular wall (vein or artery) then there is a
risk of the adherents being released into the circulation, so
after the first or second day, I would monitor alcohol intake
accordingly and discuss appropriate Vit A, D, E and
the "B" vitamin therapies with a competent physician.

Vit K is a coagulant. Chocolate likewise, successful in
stopping copious nose bleed in child in rural area.

By "adherent" I signify the anomalous teratogenic proteins i.e., rejected RNA-DNA combos sticking to arterial walls, blocking or limiting blood flow and thereby provoking the development of clots or thromboses.

Again this is not a prescription or "recommendation."
These are *not "Homeopathic" per se.*

I am sharing what I myself would do should anyone try to force these atrocities on me and Homeopathy was not available.

Other "blood thinners" or anti coagulants include cinnamon, Vitamin E, grapefruit, apple cider vinegar, etc. I mentioned tonic water, but also note that in the Pfizer catchment area Organic Tonic Water was wiped off the shelves as quickly as detergent, disinfectants and cleaning papers! Another word for Organic tonic water? Hydroxyquinine! HCQ without the chlorine!

Chocolate is a coagulant and should be avoided unless the patient is a "bleeder" or bruises easily. Cheese, milk, likewise.

At all times observe for petechiae, broken capillaries and ecchymoses, localised purple, green or yellow discoloration of patches of skin.

If the general skin tone is yellow or grey, observe for incipient or underlying liver or cardiac disease or vaccine damage.

How can I say "see a physician," even for tests when so many were killing their patients. FOR MONEY!

Purchase an OXIMETER and use it daily!

It is vital to prevent the clots from forming and the fibrins from aggregating.

Once formed, most will require surgical removal and few can afford that, even if the clots and fibrinous teratogen are discovered in time. They must be removed, even with the possibility of regrowth. Few surgeons would have the skills to safely remove these "invaders" adhering to the arterial walls.

In all cases, patients of authentic Homeopaths should continue Homeopathic protocols, to optimise recovery and prevent recurrence.

While many Homeopathic remedies have their uses in the treatment of side effects and ancillary conditions, there are just a few that might eliminate the fibrins entirely, but only for use by *skilled, expert Homeopaths. We "do surgery" without a knife, it is often said. But where we have the "invading" alien fibrins lurking on the road to the heart, we must be ultra careful.*

That being said, Homeopathy's "empathy" with the human immune system, has often surprised me, even after decades of working with Hahnemann's "miraculous" discoveries. He called Homeopathy, "The Gift of a Gracious God," a Gift he studied and used so brilliantly.

*It's interesting to note that the great "soyentists" endorsed by the CDC, NIH, etc., have finally discovered and admitted what Homeopaths have claimed for **over two centuries now,** and that is: alcoholism is a genetic condition.*

EXTREME SITUATIONS

Athletes, construction workers, pilots, distance drivers, and such, are at particular risk. Intense exercise and other stresses accelerate the heart rate, increasing the body temp and blood flow sufficiently to dislodge the alien matter, ie, the GMO/clotshot damaged fibrinogens, sending them into the heart, to block valves and kill instantly.

This is a truly tragic situation, and a physician would have to be extremely stupid and ill trained not to understand the *damage* this "experimental vaccine" would do to the population.

So the assumption is that greed, arrogance and wilful indifference to the value of human life are at the root of this genocidal substance, this "zyclon B" in a vial, and that the Nazified plan for the extermination of the human race continues apace.

But not, "a Pace!"[26]

---

[26] "apace" – rapidly. "a Pace" – to Peace!

12. <u>CURRENT MEDIA TESTIMONY:</u>

"Irish Light," Issue 10. Pfizer *knew* their "vaccines" would kill.

At first it was claimed that no animal experimentation was done.

This was followed by reports of a 100% death rate in the test creatures.

This may or may not have been the initial attempt at creating cognitive dissonance, and creating confusion and fear in a population so terrified they would comply with anything, no matter how illogical or outrageous.

1,223 deaths in the first 28 days following injection of the bioweapon.

40 Megabytes of classified info downloaded for European Medical Agency

Side Effects: Hundreds! Perhaps thousands. Pages filled with lists of post "jab" diseases and syndromes and sickness all recorded in teeny tiny illegible print, and no doubt that as many, of not many more have been redacted by the very agency funded by the taxpayers of the world to protect us from the monsters of the Islands of Dr Moreau, the Dr. Frankensteins, Mengheles, Crippens, Faucis, and Heaven knows what other upcoming young "genius" is clinging to octogenerian Fauci's lab coat tails preparing to do ultimate harm to the world at large – or their favorite targets, infants and Senior Citizens.

That is, the sadistic factor: abuse the helpless.

These side effects include: eczema, blisters, asthma, low sperm counts, and fertility problems, miscarriage (75%!) auto immunity, blindness, diabetes, herpes, cardiac problems, ie myocarditis – a very mild expression of the actual damage done by the vaccines – thyroid disorders, neuropathies, Multiple Scleroses, seizures, epilepsy, narcolepsy, Guillaine Barre Syndrome, IBS, Relapses, deafness, tongue biting, anaphylactoid syndrome of pregnancy, (ASP) anxiety, confusion, hypoxia, dyspnoea, haemorrhage and death; blood disorders, Crohn's disease and liver failure; blood clotting, (thromboses) bizarre clot formations, as in dendroids...bizarre teratological tissue formations (Dr D McN)

350 Brits died from clots post Astra Zeneca, and ecchymosis, which is interesting, if not almost contradictory – unless reversed.

This infers that the clots were not *directly* "intrinsic" to an internal deficiency or introduced toxin component.

The ecchymoses,i.e., bruising, suggests that the Astra Zeneca component[xi] contained a blood thinner, perhaps alcohol, or perhaps something I will not mention in case it gives the "ghoul school" new, inimical,ideas. Too late – they admitted snake poison!

I do not have the intel on whether the ecchymoses preceded the thromboses (clots), but I suspect that they did. It's beyond "obvious."

Ecchymoses, or bruising, are a particular vulnerability of haemophiliacs, or persons with other forms of blood deficiencies. They're also almost instantly identifiable on persons addicted to alcohol, or on blood thinners such as heparin, particularly when the dose needs "review..." i.e., is on the high side.

So, hypothetically, a "blood thinner" is introduced into the vascular system (veins and circulation) of an otherwise healthy person.

In case they *might* contract an imaginary disease from an imaginary virus.

This "blood thinner" also carries the RNA of a rodent or a macaque monkey, or the harrowed cells of an aborted baby, and the now tainted blood can distribute the lethal RNA more rapidly to the bone marrow and vital organs. *And in April 2023, it's "snake venom!"*

All the while, the mitochondrial ribosomes are busy encoding and embedding the bestial RNA with the host's inner mitochondrial membrane.

The process however, is not as "effective" as the bestial-human embryonic experiments.

Slight diversion here; these must be banned forthwith. There is absolutely no justification for these experiments. They are the product of deranged, and/or criminal minds.

When it comes to drugs, pharmadocs and pharmas are their own best customers.

In Media Res: The combination of the alien RNA and human DNA is self-limiting. As the combinations appear to start immediately in the vascular system, the tissue produced is dendritic in shape, ie, long and narrow, to fit inside the veins.

At a certain size, they block the flow of blood.

And when blood cannot flow – what does it do? How does it act?

It pools, it CLOTS. Within 7 to 10 minutes.

When the clot somehow reaches the heart – it blocks the valves, stopping the action of the heart, the circulation of the blood, the supply of oxygen to the brain and vital organs and so the patient dies.

With Anthony Fauci at the helm of the NAIAD and controlling other parties in the alphabet agencies and directing the use of mega funds for vile and unnecessary experiments such as the "covid" "virus" and "vaccines" aka BIOWEAPONS, it's not too farfetched to question whether resources were pooled, and different levels of lethality worked out between the bioweapon jab and the different pharmaceutical corporations involved in their manufacture – or even collaboration with hostile nations.

Each bioweapon / "vaccine" had its own distinct stamp or "personality."

Each functioned differently depending on age, diet, level of activity.

Some caused bizarre personality changes – most notably ModeRNA and JJ-Astra Zeneca. With Mode RNA, paranoia became striking, even in persons of formerly gentle demeanour. In one case, a "pack" mentality took over, and group behavior started to manifest – in the style of a pack of baboons, very ostensibly in one particular group; less obvious, but still apparent in others. ModeRNA contains the RNA of macaque monkeys.

I suspected the simian element, long before it was proven, by the oily black eyes in persons clearly of north European heritage. I managed to tactfully confirm that they were recently "jabbed." Babies born to "jabbed" mothers also had black oily eyes.

ModeRNA: myocarditis, pericarditis inflammation, dyspnea, apnea, paranoia – and so many, many more symptoms and anomalies.

It is very telling that the manufacturer or name of the bioweapon/jab is seldom revealed following death announcements.

I witnessed bizarre, rodent like behavior in a young woman forced to take J and J Janssen and Astra Zeneca to keep her job in the airlines. The airline only pays when the plane leaves the gate, the rest of the time she suffered alone and hungry. When invited by me to "raid" my fridge, ie, help herself, she suddenly started to behave like a drama student improvising the behavior of a rodent. Furtive movements; watchful, then scurrying... This was out of character. She was otherwise a calm, dignified young woman...

While I have no confirmation regarding the contents of these accursed bioweapons, the *public has the right to know...which animals were used in the manufacture of these lethal products.*

There was also an increase in UTI infections...as the toxic co-adjuncts passed through the ureters.

Again, there is a level of paranoia that I have witnessed in persons using ModeRNA, Pfizer and J and J, especially notable in persons where relations were long term and cordial. She seemed terrified of our gentle remedies.

Pfizer documents admit "vaccine" side effects "cause" "CV19" - a pathogen not yet proven to exist, and respiratory illness.

Pfizer was fined 4.7 *billion dollars* for false claims in the past and medical equipment *safety violations;* off label promotions; corrupt practices, kick-backs and bribery. *Prior* to the cvd scamdemic!

This should have been enough to shut them down.

After all, the Homeopaths were shut down for **superior** *statistics in our hospitals;* **superior** *survival rates;* **superior** *and prolonged recovery rates without "maintenance, ie, suppressive, medicine..."*

It is interesting to note here that the "European Union" President and arbiter of "perbenismo," i.e., middle class respectability, is married to one of Pfizer's chief executives in charge of vaccine promotion and sales.

I refer, of course, to Ursula von Leyen, daughter of Hitler's chief SS officer, Ernst Albrecht, fast tracked to the top job in Europe.

How much of a threat could a petite blonde be – without qualifications or particular talents despite attendance at several deep state, ie, far left Universities, e.g. the LSE. Sadly, the independently wealthy Ivy Leagues such as Columbia and Harvard lead the way leftward, Columbia being the wartime home of the Frankfurt School of Marxism and Harvard heavily influenced by the Sheikhs of Saudi Arabia.[27]

---

[27] Harvard's former Dean of Law, SC Judge Elena Kagan allegedly accepted $20million donation contemporaneous with the admission of

And so now, under the daughter of Hitler's No 1 henchman, Europe is once again under extreme duress, threat of genocide and under an active de-population program at great personal profit to herself, her husband and Pfizer.

Like Nazi Germany, the first to be targeted were the sick and the elderly.

However - unlike Nazi occupied Germany, there was no organised opposition from the West.

In fact, the Western powers collaborated and co-operated fully.

From the mysterious resignation of the theologically sound and recently deceased Pope Benedict XVI, the consistently "theologically" bizarre conduct of and statements by "Pope Francis I" and the collusion of the Vatican and Diocesan prelates in the idolatrous use of pathogenic masks, disinfectants, and acquiescence in the "distribution" of deadly, blasphemous, untested bioweapons, euphemistically named "vaccines," I cannot discount the possibility, even *probability* of co-operation or collaboration of P2 and the "St Gallen Mafia" in the death of millions from the toxic, inassimilable, unrecognisable, alien mRNA hybrid inventing, Pfizer, ModeRNA, J and J (Janssen) Astra Zeneca and other bioweapons aka death jabs.

After all, St. Gallen, Switzerland, is not a hundred kilometres from Davos, five minutes by air if you trust your pilot and don't fear bumping into mountains...

---

the unqualified Barack Obama to Harvard School of Law. He later appointed her to the Supreme Court of the USA.

Davos is notorious for the Bilderberg assemblies of the most greedy moguls in the history of human kind. I'm not really a Gandhi fan, but one of his quotes is here appropriate: "There is enough in this world for man's need; never enough for his greed..."

If the prelates were not willing participants in said deaths, their silence demands answers, explanations and a rational response.

Who healed lepers? Who is in the Eucharist?

Their acquiescence in the idolatrous masks, the idolatrous disinfectants, replacement of the efficacious sacramental of blessed water with alcohol gels was, from every point of view available to the Catholic practitioner and / or lay person, blasphemous!

The pathogenic mask was deemed "safer" than the author of Life, alive and ever present in the Eucharist...

The plastic bottles of disinfectant gel were regarded as having more healing power than blessed water, sacramentals, etc...? If really scared, then add a pinch of blessed, bacteriolytic salt to the blessed water!

From whom or what did they derive their information and make their decision to make the Holy Mass a nightmare...? To exclude the faithful and trusting? To allow p-harm-a controlled doctors to isolate and kill their priests and parishioners? Cui bono? Payoff?

Where were the *Catholic* MDs? Did they question the use of paralysands, of vents, of Remdesivir and the high pressure oxygen pushed into oedematous lungs?

Back to the "scientists," the experts, the sycophants who never questioned why Anthony Fauci was still leading the NIAID at the age of eighty, *despite his mercenary role in the distribution of the catastrophic AZT while young men were dying agonizing deaths from AIDS – and AZT!*

Did he have the power to remove their licences. Deny their grants? Are all physicians blackmailed? Are Homeopaths the only physicians of honor, integrity and courage?

Someone at the NIH has the power to block me from accessing material from PubMed by **lying!** They claimed I mass download their garbage. As if!!! In plain-spoke American and classic English – "Hogwash" and **they are lying!** Do I scare Foulcheat?

Who knew that li'l ole me was such a threat to the **pharm**aceutical industry aka the abortion industry, aka the organ theft industry, etc...

Aside from taking my home and stealing my proposals while NYS thugs try to assassinate me, blocking my access to professional journals is about all they can do for now.

I imagine that they could make life pretty rough for an MD that invested in their "brand" of *profiteering* health care who later saw the light, so to speak!

Something akin to standing up to *organised crime,* perhaps?

It is not as if Fauci had anything specific or helpful to say. Just wiffle waffle, ie, constantly changing the direction of the protocols, in order to deliberately create confusion and the bugbear of the 21ˢᵗ Century – **"cognitive dissonance."**

And that skill along with the "Doktah" credential was far more important to the **pharm**aceutical industry than any discardable "wonder drugs..." Just tweak a molecule or two for a new drug! Easy peasy!

And so "forked tongue" Anthony Fauci rose to the top of the Medical profession in the USA, while people dropped dead by the millions, and the drugs did their damage and were eventually recalled. A few million in compensatory damages are a "sneeze in the bucket" to the industry that makes BILLIONS off each new "wonder drug" aka "magic pill and is licensed to generate new customers every single day by injecting vials of toxins into the arms of little babies...or distributing mifipristone abortion drug (RU 486) into the internal organs of expecting mothers.

No warning, of course, of the risk of miscarriage in their living room or that they might haemorrhage to death alone like a young woman in France, seeing her dead, bloodied, baby as the light left her eyes.

Not a problem to "one size fits all" medicine for marketing!

So welcome to a world where humanity is divided every which way... into sexual preferences, bizarre self mis-identifications, Generations, Boomers, Gen X, Y, Z, Zoomers...etc., *mothers against their pre-natal infants.*

Division weakens. In unity there is strength.

Why does "Gen Z" coincide with the timing of the **genocidal intent of the "covid 19" scamdemic and the subsequent artificially generated panic, fear and terror,**

---

28 Except there is some debate re the mass suicides of lemmings!

and mass hysteria - driving humanity to the death jabs, like lemmings[28] over a cliff. "Z" is the last letter of the alphabet. Is "Gen Z" supposed to be the last *fully human* generation?

If not, why did trained chemists, biologists, pharmacists and medical professionals, acquiesce in such a vile and **predictably homicidal practice. As "Deep Throat" notoriously stated: "Follow the Money!"**

The Hippocratic Oath was discarded in 1973 at the time when it became fashionable and lucrative to murder babies in utero. The lowered birth rate combined with the feminist movement shaming mothers out of the home and into the work force more or less doubled the supply of workers. This allowed for lower salaries, fewer benefits and, with IT, increased reliance on part time workers.

MDs no longer promise to "First Do No Harm!"

Since 1973 many have "done" serious harm to their patients. A cynicism has crept in along with a computerised mockery of the doctor-patient relationship and increased reliance on "technicians."

The human "corpus" is now divided and subdivided *ad absurdum* to the point where we are more or less divided into a bunch of cytoplasmic substrates, about whose immediate functions the "soyentists" can expound *ad nauseum* but about whose ultimate role they understand little or nothing.

Something like our kindly friends in IT driving the world off the AI cliff in an exquisitely designed "vehicle" without any comprehension as to the need for brakes – or the ultimate consequences...

...of letting robots control humanity.

They might be even worse than Fauci, Redfield, Ghebyrous &Co. Perish that thought!

They not only "do harm," but are indifferent to the ultimate result of the replication of the harm that they do.

The ultimate in sociopathy!

"April 2023 <thegreatclimatecon.com>

MONTANA LEGISLATION. COVID BILL 645

CRIMINALISES DONATION OF BLOOD OR TISSUE FROM "COVID" VACCINATED PERSONS."

AFTER THAT BILL IS PASSED, WILL THE EVIDENCE BE AVAILABLE TO INDICT FAUCI, GATES, REDFIELD, BIRX, DRAGHI, XI JING PING AND ALL CONCERNED AT UNC, WUHAN, NEW CHINA, Lombardy, FOR CRIMES AGAINST HUMANITY?

13. FIRST DO NO HARM – HIPPOCRATIC OATH

Most people today, educated or not, appear to believe that the Hippocratic Oath is still administered to all qualifying physicians.

Interestingly the licensed slaughter of babies in God's "safest of all places"[29] followed the first cardiac transplants by the South African doctors... Even though their patients did not survive well, transplants suddenly became the new diamond mine for the Pharmaceutical, Medical and Surgical divisions of so called "Health care."

And the big secret to the "success" of the transplant injury came from China: the use of **organs removed from living political prisoners – proned and paralysed!**

This would "never be accepted" in the United States, not even if applied to mass murderers.

*But throw in a few word games, such as "brain dead," and hey presto, everyone is running to register themselves on their drivers' licenses as **organ donors.***

How virtuous.

How horrifying!

Brief, succinct...a con job based on "brain dead..."

Not so "brain dead" as to feel every single cut of the surgeons' scalpels as they cut into and remove every organ one by one by one.

---

[29] Rabid atheists may be tempered by the use of the words: "Nature's safe place..." ignoring, of course, that Nature is God's Creation!

The "PPP" protocol: the patient proned and paralysed, as pressurised oxygen is forced into damaged lungs, penetrating the tissue and killing the patient slowly while the organs are removed from his/her body, while the patient weeps in agony and helplessness.

This is one of the most sadistic of all murders. By Medical Doctors and nurses.

A **horror story** that continues to this day.

While the world looks away.

Then again, they kill babies, don't they? So cruel, so sadistic, so vile is abortion. THERE IS NO RIGHT TO MURDER ANOTHER HUMAN PERSON.

Why were organs needed so desperately in 20/21/22?

So desperately, that cities run by the Democrat Party, in bed with China's Jing Ping and the Soros-Schwab cartel, devised a vicious ideology for removing organs from Senior Citizens and anyone presenting with anything as "lethal" as an ingrown toenail.

But I exaggerate there. Just a bit.

A certain front for special interests, once originating in Mongolia...and entering the Western, European nations through lies and deception, and faking membership in one of the world's "Abrahamic" religions, worked every angle possible to terrify the public into believing that *proning* patients with dyspnea, apnea or other forms of respiratory distress was a good idea.

It is cruel and inhuman to force a patient with respiratory distress to lie face down on his or her abdomen, blocking the free action of the "diaphragm" which functions as a sort of "bellows" regulating the action of the lungs...

It does, however, facilitate organ removal, China style...leaving the beating heart to the last...

They didn't mention that this is the first step in the removal of organs.

As most of medical – **pharm**aceutical victims were healthy, with minor issues, Remdesevir was added to the lethal protocol. This I discovered post facto.

Remdesivir damages the kidneys, leading to oedema/edema, bloating, swelling of limbs and lungs...preparing them for the ultimate *"coup de grace."*[30]

Then when the patient is sufficiently weakened, or at any time an unethical physician chooses, a ventilator is inserted into the carotid artery...

The ventilator was attached to a machine which could raise or lower the pressure at any time.

At the "appropriate" time, paralysands are administered and the ventilator pressure increased to the point where the damaged lungs are punctured by the concentrated air stream. Secret autopsies in Italy and the USA revealed HOLES in the lungs of persons allegedly treated in hospitals and nursing homes for "Covid."

The paralysands are used to keep the patient still while he or she suffers indescribable agony as his or her organs are

---

[30] Torture of Catholics, etc., in medieval times was often followed by beheading, the "blow of grace," ie ended the torture, so a "good thing...???"

removed, one by one, or in the case of the kidneys, two by two. No anaesthetics are required.

Wasn't there a "kinder, gentler" method of mass murder?

Actually, the mass murderer, being a demonically - possessed psychopath by definition, will choose the most painful and ignominious death for his/her victims...and, in that kind, perpetrators of vaccines – people like Bill Gates and his protectors, Mark Zuckerberg, etc., will work to inflict the maximum suffering possible on human kind – their brothers and sisters on this planet.

Gates was charged with genocide in India, tried – in absentia, his own choice – convicted and sentenced to execution.

He will never visit India again.

Similarly Africa, but the President of the small nation which charged him was murdered.

Just coincidentally, after taking tea with Susan Rice...

14. **RATIONALES**

For example: "We didn't know it would kill. We just wanted the money."

Those who openly opposed the lies re "covid" and exposed the murders that occurred in hospitals and and nursing homes, and warned emphatically about the "fake-zines" ie death jabs, "Zyclon B" in a vial, those honest professionals were harassed, hounded, and we suspect that some were murdered.

https://twitter.com/michael.../status/13995838883352 69889...

For instance, the inventor of the PCR test, Kary Mullis, warned about the abuse of said test by Fauci in the 1980s. https://www.tabletmag.com/.../articles/masked-ball-cowardice .

Kary Mullis died mysteriously in August of 2019.

August seems to be a popular time for the deep state's "dirty deeds..." The world is relaxed after the summer vacations, but focused on "back to work, kids to school," etc., so little attention is paid to such pivotal events as the sudden death of a health 74 year old Nobel Prize scientist, the arch enemy of "soy-entist" Anthony Fauci.

There are many reports of the death of Kary Mullis online. The link below best represents public opinion, or at least the opinion of members of the public most invested in truth.

Others have died or been silenced.

I survived two attempts on my life in 2006 when my proposal to continue to use Homeopathy to wean long term patients was "stolen" by the Medical Director of the Hospital, in conjunction with Langone and NYU. It passed six committees and vanished! "Fauci's orders?"

I naively rented an apartment in Pfizer territory but was unlawfully evicted by perjured testimony. It took the collusion of three corrupt "judge magistrates" and a travesty of a hearing. The corrupt judge did not allow me to refute aforesaid perjuries. Even more farcical, he ordered *all mention of the existence of contrary evidence,* i.e., my *supporting* evidence, to be wiped from the records. His name is James Gallagher and he "presides" in Bryn Mawr. His primary cohort was Francis Lawrence of the notoriously corrupt Norristown Court system.

*In fact, anyone convicted or evicted in those courts should have their records completely expunged, their fines returned and liberties restored, indisputable violent crimes excepted. Every case that came before Gallagher and Lawrence should be immediately nullified. That is how deep the corruption goes, corruption which I witnessed and experienced for the "crime" of **saving lives in the time of "covid."***

At that time my "covid" patients enjoyed a 24-72 hour full recovery rate. Their symptoms corresponded to vaccinoses from the 2019 flu vax and or contact with recently vaccinated persons shedding the more virulent elements of the vaccine – coughing, sneezing, "tactile" exchange... eg perspiration, bodily fluids, etc.

It is my opinion, again as yet uncorroborated, that the 2019 flu shot contained rodent mRNA. It would not be beyond the grossly unethical "sci-bots" at Pfizer to release their infected rodents into public areas.

Just a tiny bit kinder than playing "Jai Alai" with the artificially sickened creatures, i.e., smashing their tortured bodies against the walls or dropping living rodents into the grinders and watching them being shredded alive - as described by an eye-witness who now hates all furry creatures after working at Pfizer.

Guilt.

As I said – psychopaths.[31]

And we trust them with our health, our care, our lives???

---

[31] The psychopath takes pleasure in the suffering of others. The "sociopath" is indifferent, concerned only with his / her satisfaction, ambition, pleasure.

15. MEDIA RES – *Heart of the Matter*

My initial reaction to reading the contents of the so called "covid" "vaccines" was one of profound HORROR!

Even with my skills and experience as a Homeopath, The mRNA would be a nightmare. It would not be analogous to anti-doting a toxin, or precisely stimulating the immune system toward a specific response, but would require careful analyses, a deep knowledge of our remedies, precise report of symptoms from the patient and patient's family, possible recourse to unusual protocols, and *no interference* from outside "medications." And patience!

That would be "NO REMDESIVIR!" Not ever!

This is all over the head of the "Old School" Medicine, and we can see from their response to the effects of the "deathjab" that they have no authentic scientific response. They are baffled and now throwing, guess what, all the alternative and once despised "hippy" medicines of the despised "holistic" school at these teratogenic products. Said products are the result of introducing **bestial RNA into the bloodstreams, hence *recombining* with the DNA of living human persons.**

But not Homeopathy, because they are clueless.

Said "products" *won't go away* and just keep killing people.

Not only that, but the vicious teratogenic tissue keeps replicating and **"recombining"** until it clogs the veins and arteries, blocking the flow of blood or attaches to tissue, limiting blood flow, thereby facilitating the formation of... static blood clots!

Static blood clots within 7 minutes. Haemophiliacs excepted.

If the teratogenic tissue is sufficiently narrow to allow a shallow flow of blood, and if it is adherent to a vascular wall (vein or artery) the patient will still function, but with difficulty, eg, suffer from hypoxia, headaches, fatigue, eyestrain, etc.

When an athlete is on the field, the excess temperatures generated by intense, competitive activity cause the tissues and vascular system to expand. The heart rate increases, the blood pressure, rises putting pressure on the alien tissue, forcibly separating from the vascular wall and releasing it into the bloodstream, thereby directly into the heart.

If not the dendritic teratogens, then the clots.

If the blood cannot flow, it will clot,

So, liquid blood, blocked and unable to flow into the heart and thence to lungs to dump carbon dioxide (CO2) and pick up oxygen, will simply pool and clot behind the blockage.

Clever little homicidal strategy.

All deaths, of course, by "natural causes."

Challenge: Convince me that your top MDs didn't anticipate this, even with the deficiencies in the medicine of the "ghoul school."[32]

I am both a serious, world class dramatist and a Homeopath.

Both disciplines give us laser sharp insight into human behavior, social and emotional in the case of drama, and pathological, cognitive and bio-emotional where Homeopathy is most informative. But it does take ethics, even faith in the Creator to be a good Homeopath. Because it is a challenge. Each patient is unique – differing levels of energy, different aetiologies, e.g., genetic, lifestyle, nutritional intake or absences, environmental...all of vital interest.

The sniggering, smirking, sneering behavior of Fauci, Gates, Birx, Redfield, et al, mark them as "members" of a private "club" or "clique," or "claque!" A "claque," that is crude and indifferent to human suffering.

They are "in" on a secret which cannot be shared with the general public, a secret which allows them to snigger and smirk in private – or, realistically speaking, as soon as the press conferences end.

What secret? Sales of human organs? "Vaccine" targets? Genocide? Mega sums of money purloined from the taxpayer?

------

[32] Reference does not include the few remaining, dedicated, ethical, "old school" physicians who appear to have ceased practice rather than continue with this farce. They were trained as *physicians*, not "technicians,"and many "resigned" during the scam.

In working with and having access to RNA research, they *must* have witnessed the worst atrocities and abuses of Crick, Watson and Rosemary Franklin's discoveries.

Remember Rosemary?

Of course not! Dr. Franklin was the female intelligence behind the discovery of helical DNA and so was "buried" in the annals of history, somewhere between "Frankfurter" and "Frankenstein."

All Hail Crick and Watson! (sarcasm) *"Cherchez la femme?"* In the field of science, yes, look for the woman concealed behind the discoveries. In this context, the woman is solution – *not* the problem, at least until she demands recognition and recompense.

Back to "worst possible uses..." The transhumanist agenda... the splicing of rodent[33] and human embryos, or cerebral tissue (pfizer)the splicing of leporiditae RNA with human DNA and other diabolical exercises have led to the most vile and intolerable results, beyond even the wildest fantasies of Dr Moreau and the screenwriters of "Star Wars," etc. "Hybridised" humans.

It is interesting that Hollywood "tips us off" in terms of impending atrocities, bragging, daring us to see through them!

However, such movies are usually so far ahead of contemporary lunacies that they are quickly dismissed as fantasy, or science fiction when, in fact, they are

---

[33] Rodent – rats, mice, guinea pigs, etc. Leporiditae – rabbits.

"conditioning" films for the naïve or resistant. Thus the instigators mock our naivete even more intensely.

Would abortion have been accepted or tolerated without "Omen," "Damien," "Children of the Corn," and the umpteen self-pitying, "poor me" story lines of mid to upper income women well supported by their spouses, but suddenly deciding, after having five children, that it's time to return to law school and let the little ones get themselves off to school and take over the chores etc. One NY Times Mag article *celebrated* a *five year old* child who set his alarm, readied his clothes at night, got up unprompted and unassisted in the morning, prepared breakfast and school lunch and got himself out to school. Role reversal. Nauseating.

Children may be capable of extraordinary resilience and diligence e.g., the savage world is full of exploited, capable child workers, but that is the *contradiction* of childhood – ideally a time of imagination and wonder, cherishing, emotional cocooning and safety.

NY Times had a slew of "child as parent or self-parent" stories, to which it added a "charming" (sarcasm) item on a Chinese female pediatrician's favorite dish – potage au enfant abortee! Baby embryo soup.

Yes, in the supposedly prestigious New York Times!

Crickets. Not a word of outrage.

Job done.

And so, over the deadly cliff of transhumanism we humans are driven!

Whatever happened to critical thinking? Whatever happened to reason, analyses, ethics?

*"Bioethics" is a travesty, imo. Not worth the paper it's printed on. A well-funded "study" for the purpose of manipulating the public into believe that "ethics" is synonymous with **ethical! No it is not! It's a "buyable" principle.***

Millions paying off tens of thousands in college debt and they don't even know how to think for themselves. Or where to start.

America's Founding Fathers churning in their graves!

16. FACING DOWN THE RNA

RNA is not "inert."[34] At the right temperature[35] it is alive and active, and ready to combine and recombine ad infinitum with any other available RNA or DNA.

In the wrong corpus it is a ticking time bomb. *Every human "corpus" is the wrong corpus for bestial RNA!*

In other words, it is highly unstable at temps above minus 80 degrees Fahrenheit and will grab onto any unstable ribosome waving in its direction...

The following link[36], found after I wrote this reveals the depths of depravity associated with Transhumanism and the most degenerate of humans who try to impose it on the world. Other links which I shall "end note"[xii] expose the most unconscionable, vile, disgusting, immoral experiments in what is now called Transhumanism.

"Transhumanism" is a euphemism for the most evil "research" of the "Fauci" school of "soyence," ie, Science in the Service of Sa+an.

Science is the study of Creation, and the best use to make of the Gifts given to the children of the Lost Paradise.

---

[34] https://medicine.iu.edu/faculty-labs/corson/protocols/rna-precautions
[35] Comfortable at - 80 degrees fahrenheit.
[36] https://theimaginativeconservative.org/2021/05/jeffrey-epstein-hideous-strength-transhumanism-joseph-pearce.html#respond

"Soy-ence" is man's arrogant desire to replace God (as if!) and doom the world time and time again. Whenever humankind reaches a homeostasis or healthy, pleasant balance, in come the "soy-entists" and mess it up again...in consort with corrupt politicians, ie snakes and their venom makers – pharmakopeia....

I will note here, that Paradise, aka Eden, was lost due to the jealousy and control issues of a female, manipulated by an envious "serpent!" And those chomping on the forbidden apples of DNA and RNA doom us time and again. On the other hand,"Blokey"[37] Adam was quite content with his companion and pretty garden and talking creatures.

Not to feed the misogynists, but Eve's motivation in taking the forbidden apple from the Tree of Knowledge was to acquire knowledge and power attributable to, accessible by, God alone.

The most offensive "knowledge" sought may have been "power" over life and death. Like Fauci &Co with their delves into genetic recombinants.

And thereby hangs a grim tale as they "follow the minotaur" into and around and around a labyrinth with neither exit nor return.

Genetics *qua* orthodox or standardised science is a fractalian exercise, one substrate breaking off into

---

[37] "Bloke" is an English (UK) term for a gentle man content with family, Faith and a down to earth lifestyle. Gentle, but strong.

another and yet another, until the original intent and knowledge vanishes or appears obsolete. Like the branches of a tree that become increasingly fragile the farther they grow from their soil and source.

As a Classical Homeopath, working with the original and unique "genetic therapy" developed by the genius of the 18th Century, I am shocked at the primitiveness of the concept behind the "Covid" "vaccine," aka **bioweapon,** that is, bestial mRNA concealed within a trojan horse of toxins and pathogens designed with the purpose of confusing and blindsiding the sophisticated and awesome strategies of the human immune system to the point where, "confused" it goes into "overdrive" setting up the patient to appear seriously ill, or dying, thus providing a rationale for admitting said patient to hospital where Remdesivir and the vent could cruelly and savagely end their lives – Remdesivir by destroying the kidneys, causing pulmonary oedema and the vent to puncture the lungs with high pressure oxygen.

It is also shocking to consider how many science departments, in high schools and University science faculties – including those serving Med Schools **failed** to call "Big p-harm-a to account, or even question their concepts, strategies and statistics.

Then again, follow the money!

Each "death with Covid corpse" = $50k to $200k.

Is academia prostituting itself to the p*harm*aceutical industry? Is DC? More to the point – what State, politician, educational establishment, etc., is *not!*

Power is a dangerous beast. Over centuries its abuse has led to the slaughter of hundreds of millions of innocent people.

And now the Fauxcis, Gates, Birxes of this world and cohorts are engaged in homicidal research. That is, experiments which are not only repulsive and sickening when performed on innocent creatures but intensely dangerous to human Life. *Homicidal!*

It is increasingly apparent, even proven by recently released US Defense Department Documents, that the intent was to destroy human life **on an unprecedented scale – unprecedented even by Nazi and Stalinist standards.**[38]

Given that a certain banking cartel, notorious for its globalist outreach, is run by descendants of the notorious, highly organised but ruthless and blood thirsty Genghis Khan, and has infiltrated the highest echelons of government in Europe, Asia, Australia and the USA, the time has come for an intense prayer crusade and strong, ethical, political and spiritual leadership.

We are on the brink, indeed, are dangling over the edge of a cliff, looking downward at jagged rocks marked "WEF," "NOW," "UN," "WHO" as so called leaders sign their nations into the most malevolent dictatorship since the Aztecs.[39]

---

[38] https://twitter.com/SpartaJustice/status/1631549284402200576

In other words, democracy is in extreme danger of extinction. No easier conquest than a population dependent on psychotropes.

Except a fourth generation damaged by and dependent on psychotropes. "Recreational" drugs by any other name destroy cognitive function.

Does this reflect the terrifying lack of control of and "obeisance" to the p-harm-aceutical industry by Government agencies mandated to monitor and "contain" them?

Have they become the *de facto* government of the USA, and other nations?

Or the enablers of despotism?

They are allowed to produce and distribute one harmful product after another until their evident dangers and damage to the population lead to product recall, too often after the patent expires and billions of dollars are tucked away in their vaults or private accounts.

And then they claim more public funds for research. Obscene.

Profit or power?

Whatever their motivation, the lack of any oversight is terrifying. An industry invested in bio-weapon research and profiteering from disease and human

---

[39] Sacrificed up to 12,000 innocents per day by tearing out their hearts.

suffering must not be allowed to function without oversight and accountability.

Better yet, **shut down completely!**

The mRNA loaded "vaccines" – *de facto* bioweapons distributed intensely and relentlessly to innocent, trusting, naïve persons around the globe demonstrate that that "Big *pharma" is totally *out of control.*

It is no longer "attached to the "arterial wall," that is, any form of control: it has broken free and is heading to the all too trusting heart of humanity for another attempt at a "Final Solution."

17. "GENETICS" – CUI BONO?

<u>https://duckduckgo.com/?q=splicing+human+and+ani</u>
<u>mal+dna&t=ffab&atb=v222-1&ia=web</u>

The above search link exposed some of the most vile "experiments" imagineable, including the "product" of combining animal RNA with Human DNA… in one photo a creature that was of both human and rodent (rabbit) origin. I saw the "frog child" over a decade ago. It took almost a decade to get those tragic images out of my mind.

Are they human? Do we baptise them?

These, and the other links clarify the aetiology of the smug smirks of the "nerds," eg Fauci, Gates, Zuckerman, and probably thousands of other "soyentists" around the world, most notably in UNC,[40] USA and Wuhan, China.

I would not be in the least surprised if the "transhuman" bio-spliced creatures were also "developed" in the Ukraine bioweapons laboratories target bombed by Vladimir Putin.

They're "in" on a huge private "joke" which they intend to impose on and have partly pulled on a naïve and trusting world. In this they are aided and abetted by celebrities and sycophants, many of which are set up for blackmail at the onset of their careers. To keep them

---

[40] University of North Carolina, where Fauci allegedly oversaw the development of a "rigged" 2019 flu vaccine which he then sent to Wuhan for mass production. It was not as lethal as expected.

in line and allow their "use" as "spokespersons" or "exemplars" for the "deep state," i.e., covert thieves of power.

The smirk inducing "joke" includes adrenochrome, taken from the corpse of torture victims, child trafficking, organ theft, iatrogenic murder, etc., and other serious crimes against Humanity. In all there appears to be a profound hatred of babies and children, i.e., hatred of Creation, of life itself, of God.

Great discoveries were made by men and women of Faith.

The most destructive abuses of Creation were made by "soy-entists," arrogant creatures attempting to usurp God. Like the serpent mentioned earlier.

Hollywood demands constant attention and awareness. Not only do their movies alert us to the future plans of the "deep state" "soyentists," they also provide blueprints, ie plans of action, etc., to the socially awkward "nerds" determined to sink humanity to the bestial level of Star Wars, ie, a world of Wookies and Jabbas and R2D2s, etc... "Diversity" amplified.

Because, quite frankly, that seems to be the direction if not the exact plan.

When I see "Marty," the giant, "friendly" robot scooting about Giant Supermarket, it seems only a matter of a brief space in time when he will be *weaponised* and we will be "commanded" or "dropped" by those heartless machines, cute though they have been made to appear with large eyes, and smiley faces, etc., for now! *"Get into line six or be zapped..."*

"Line six" being the line to, say, the carbon monoxide enabled trucks used by the Turks to murder the Armenians.

The ATMS, the Self Service Check out, the Cell Phones, the digital age, the "hey presto" here's a bitcoin, etc., *none for our benefit.*

All to reduce service, maximise profit, demean humanity.

Neither is State funded research.

Why do profiteering corporations ask for Federal Funding? Why do they receive it? Cui bono?

Our lads and lassies in the military?

The Statemust cease and desist forthwith from funding private mega buck corporations.

More trenchantly, the "State" must also keep a close eye on pharmaceutical research promulgated in major Universities, especially the power hungry Ivy Leagues.

Taxpayer funded watchdog agencies failed drastically, criminally, to protect the American public. They must be held accountable and removed from any dialogue with the pharma**s. Social media blocked all persons and expressions of concern.**

I repeat once more: we already have a Divinely Inspired, deeply and authentically scientific protocol for the cure, repeat, *cure,* of disease and that is, authentic Homeopathy. *Again, authentic* Homeopathy, the most advanced healing protocol in the world.

18. BEHAVIORAL CHANGES

There is neither excuse nor explanation for the use of the so called anti covid "vaccines."

These are neither "vaccines" nor gene "therapy."

There is nothing "therapeutic" about the contents of the "vaccines," neither in theory, intent, nor practice.

Crick and Watson have a lot to answer for.

Gene splicing has been used to add, say, fish flounder genes to tomatoes to keep them fresh longer.

Seriously? More from the weird mind of Dr. F?

There are also terrifying videos from secret laboratories, apparently in East Europe, where transhumanism is practiced – apparently from an embryonic level, the results of which are heartbreaking.

DNA and RNA in the hands of monsters are then used, not as "therapy" but as *weapons*, to create more monsters or kill the normal, intelligent members of the human species.

Pfizer has not revealed the bestial source of the RNA used in its death jabs. Rumor suggests scorpions, rats, canines, etc., and circa March-April 2023, some covert source came up with snake venom. How appropriate! Mode RNA uses Macaque monkeys, which I knew about before it became public...just by observing the effects on persons who had recently taken it.

I first witnessed it in the watery, almost oily BLACK eyes in pale Euro-Americans, in the Southern US States. They were probably already contaminated in the North East USA, but I was unable to stay and observe.

I also noted animalistic behavior in the recently jabbed in NE USA, and later, in Italy. People once considered as kindly friends, started to behave like a pack of baboons – or macaques. Scientific interest vs fear!!!

I have seen rodent type movements and conduct in a person who took J and J aka Janssen, and Astra Zeneca – who was also subjected to considerable, intense UTIs, a very sweet young lady, who left soon after, so no follow up.

The UTIs may have been one of the body's eliminative systems compromised or confused by perhaps another alien component or bioweapon.

As Pfizer may have intended if it were their people who forced me out of PA and into a nomadic existence.

There is neither justification nor rationale for what was done to me and my family in Norristown and Bryn Mawr, PA, USA i.e. "Pfizer-GSK country!"

In other words, not only kill the patients, but destroy those with the greatest possibility of saving their lives.

So, yes, Genocide.

And yes, the personality changes continue, people becomingly depressed, or – aggressive and animalistic! And dying, dropping dead in front of our eyes as the clots "unlatch," and clog the heart.

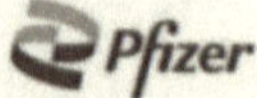

Global Product Development

06 May 2021

Marion Gruber, Ph.D.
Director
Office of Vaccines Research and Review
Food and Drug Administration
Center for Biologics Evaluation and Research
Document Control Center
10903 New Hampshire Avenue
WO71, G112
Silver Spring, MD 20993-0002

Re: **BLA 125742**

      COVID-19 mRNA Vaccine (BNT162/PF-07302048)

      Part 1 of the Original Submission – Rolling Biologics License Application (BLA)

      Request for Priority Review Designation

Dear Dr. Gruber,

Please find enclosed Part 1 of the Original Submission of the rolling Biologics License Application (BLA) for the BNT162b2 vaccine candidate developed by BioNTech and Pfizer under BB-IND 19736 for the prevention of COVID-19 caused by SARS-CoV-2 in individuals ≥16 years of age. This vaccine was granted Fast Track Designation for individuals ≥18 years of age on 07 July 2020. The Grant Fast Track Designation Letter is provided in Module 1.7.4. Submission of this BLA as a rolling application was agreed during the teleconference of 16 April 2021.

BioNTech and Pfizer are requesting Priority Review Designation for this BLA. It meets the criteria for Priority Review Designation, as outlined in the 2014 *Guidance for Industry: Expedited Programs for Serious Conditions – Drugs and Biologics* because BNT162b2 prevents a serious and life-threatening condition (COVID-19) and, if approved, would provide a significant improvement in safety and effectiveness because there are currently no vaccines licensed for the prevention of COVID-19 in the US. The Priority Review Designation Request is provided in Module 1.2.

A wire transfer for $2,875,842.00 was made to the U.S. Department of Treasury (TREAS

19. CAUSATIVE FACTORS IN SUDDEN DEATH and MITIGATION OF mRNA BIOWEAPONS.

It is almost self-evident, from the "clots" and bizarre tissue formations removed from the corpses of those who died following "vaccine" usage, that the alien or bestial RNA contained within the "vaccines" *cannot safely or effectively* combine with the DNA of the mature human. Instead of creating a viable life form, as occurs with the most revolting and repulsive of embryonic bestial-human experimental "transcriptions," teratological protein forms start developing, alerting the immune system to the necessity for intense response. The body then goes into hyper-drive in its attempts to eliminate the teratogen or damaged product from its vascular system.

Heart rate accelerates, blood pressure elevates, epinephrines flood into the system along with white blood cells, leukocytes, and T4, T8 carrying lymphocytes etc....

Two things occur... the tissue formed by the RNA-DNA **blocks** the circulation of the blood, and so it pools and thereby **clots.**

The clot either "sidesteps" the blockage and is ported directly to the heart, or it simply stops the flow of blood to the heart.

Either way, life stops. Patient is dead. Resuscitation almost impossible, due to the blockages. This is the most likely outcome for the older or more sedentary populations.

Where athletes are concerned, they are in good physical shape and so can maintain activity, albeit not at the same level as (relatively) pureblooded, i.e., before the death*jabs and with more "minor" adversities, e.g., headaches, pain, etc.   When their activity is accelerated, the body's temperature, T, rises, the Blood Pressure increases, and so increased pressure is applied to the "tissue" obstructions (protein) clinging to the veins or arteries. They cannot withstand the pressure and so the alien proteins are pushed into circulation, thence directly into the heart or brain, blocking valves and vasculars, i.e., veins, arteries and capillaries, thereby ending life.

Heightened body temperature is a factor here, also, as the RNA functions best at cooler temperatures, and so starts to degrade, diminishing density and tenacity.

Death ensues.

The multiplicity of symptoms and corporeal changes found in the bodies of those who were "up to code" with vaccines, i.e., fully "vaxed" suggest that the human immune system engaged in all out, full on biological **warfare** against the invading substances.

"Warfare" that would have been largely successful were the body just combatting "simple" poison.

HOW DARE Fauci, Jing, Birx, Draghi, the Irish Health Services, the Alphabet, ie "DEEP STATE," "protective" health monitoring agencies, allow this travesty, this irreversible toxin, this "zyclon b in a syringe" to be promulgated and used around the world against millions of naïve and trusting people.

It is impossible to comprehend, excuse or endorse at *any level under any circumstances.*

Impossible! No excuse whatsoever for inserting the RNA of simian, rodent, and Heaven alone knows what other species, into the bloodstreams of innocent, trusting, naïve, ill-informed human persons...PREGNANT WOMEN, and LITTLE CHILDREN.

We do not need any more "**Monsters.**" We have them already. They are **Pfizer, ModeRNA, Janssen (j and j) GSK, Astra Zeneca, and those who enabled them, Ursula von Leyen and her Pfizer vaks sales husband, of the EU: Fauci; Birx: Redfield: Biden-Obama: Pelosi: Jing: Draghi: Senior members of the CDC, NIH, FDA, NIAID, Wuhan Labs, UNC,** etc, etc, ad nauseum.

Sad to say, allegedly also some officials in the US Department of Defense.

20. POTENTIAL PROTOCOLS.

Homeopathic potentials are colloquially termed "remedies." Keeps it simple.

However, the correct term is "potential."

Because until the "remedy" meets the "totality of symptoms" resonating within a patient, it is a potential.

If the resonance is not precise, the immune system will ignore it.

Solutions:

As Homeopathy is exacting and precise it is difficult to give general recommendations without knowing the patient and his/her exact symptoms and concomitants.

These may be better administered after the following:

While hemorrhage is not unknown among "vaccine" victims, the majority of reports relate to clots, clots, more clots, and bizarre tissue formations.

Isolated RNA does not thrive in heat nor alcohol.

Therefore, generally speaking, if a deathjab were forced on me - **Heaven forbid!** - my very first action would be the immediate ingestion of a hot whiskey with water and cinnamon. All are anti coagulants.

For alcoholics, or persons sensitive too or with religious objections to alcohol, apple juice or apple cider vinegar may offer a close substitute, again with cinnamon, turmeric, Vitamins A, D, E – in appropriate strengths. Pinch of cinnamon in warm water can also be beneficial if taken immediately following a coerced or regretted shot, but *do consult a knowledgeable health professional, preferable one who already knows and understands your health status.*

For those with a more haemorrhagic diathesis, HOT CHOCOLATE provides warmth to assist in the breakdown of the mitrochondria and is an excellent, emergency, coagulant. Chocolate can also be efficacious in nosebleeds, etc., and isn't spoiled too badly by the addition of cinnamon.

There are Homeopathic remedies for the haemorrhagic constitutions but they should only be used by experienced Homeopaths, and certainly never fall into the malevolent minds and hands of the **harma**ceutical industry.

Too many people across the USA are mis-using our amazing "potentials" aka "remedies." Diabolically clever of the **pharm**a industry to take over the "natural health" movement and dump our incredible, precise and demanding protocols on the shelf with the "mushroom teas..." metaphorically speaking.

As a result thousands of persons believe they have "tried" Homeopathy when, in fact, they have simply misused a remedy, inappropriately.

I don't know if Boericke and Tafel, the great Philadelphia Homeopathic Pharmacy was forced to close or couldn't take the competition from Boiron, which mainstreamed remedies with a uni-symptom use stamped on their tubes.

Their product is excellent, but they do Homeopathy no favors with this approach.

We prescribe according to the *totality of the symptoms,* and monitor progress closely, but not to the point of distraction or obsession. That is counter-productive.

With the headway that I made, we would be practicing in the hospitals, healing and restoring life and hope to the sickest of the sick.

But that was sabotaged.

There are perhaps ten remedies with possible direct application for the resorption of the alien proteins.

The dedicated student of Homeopathy might recognise the remedies from the briefest of descriptions, but as I have not yet had the opportunity to treat the post "vaccination" population, speculation would not here be appropriate.

And it would be disastrous if they were to fall into the clutches of the **pharm**aceutical industry and their cohorts in DC.

21. ABOUT HOMEOPATHY

Homeopathy is the most refined and sophisticated therapeutic protocol of all time. It's efficacy is a threat to those who would profiteer from the sickness and suffering of others.

While we are grateful for and deeply respect the work of the monastic and genuine herbalists, our direct origins are rooted in a bark discovered by a Catholic Saint and Surgeon, one St. Martin de Porres, OP, and sent to Europe from Peru, via Jesuit missionaries.

He called it Cinchona Bark after the Countess of Cinchon, in gratitude to her generosity to the poor.

Some centuries later, it reached the laboratory of one Dr. Samuel Hahnemann, physician and pharmacist of Leipzig under the adapted name of "Quinine."

Yes, the same "Quinine" in tonic water!

Hahnemann noted that the symptoms displayed by a very sick friend were almost identical to those induced by excess consumption of Quinine or "tonic water," and so developed and proven time and time again, the LAW of Similars.

That which causes illness in material quantities cures the same illness in micro-diluted and succussed or dynamised quantities. LET LIKES CURE LIKE!!!

Galen and Hippocrates had both touched on the theory of "Similia Similibus Curentur" a nod to the Doctrine of Similars whereby a plant's color and shape can reveal the purpose for which the Lord designed it.

This has held true for the herbalists and Homeopaths to the present day, even pharma meds adhering to some of those discoveries.

For example, purple plants such as foxglove were noted to be effective when used for a heart condition, weakness or failure. Extract of foxglove is now called "digitalis," and is synthesised by the pharma industry – which pays no royalties to the herbalists of yore, nor to their descendants, just sabotages us at every turn.

Yellow plants are associated with bile and the liver.

One of the most outstanding is the pre-eminent, amazing, powerful, therapeutic but despised DANDELION!

Back to Hahnemann and Quinine. The great Doctor Hahnemann administered quinine to his friend who started to recover almost immediately.

That was probably the first time Quinine was used for Malaria, as the symptoms are suggestive of Malaria, although details are scarce.

From there on, Hahnemann and dedicated colleagues embarked on the most intense and dedicated study of the causative symptoms and curative properties of every substance on God's great earth, from plants and herbs, to animal and insect venoms, to elements and compounds, but dilute and dynamised!

The active ingredient in Hydroxychloroquinine sulphate is Quinine, one of the few helpful allopathic products during the "Covid 19" scare, ie, when fear and terror aggravated the effects of a "doctored" 2019 flu vaccine.

My suspicions tended toward contamination with rodent spittle, mucus or DNA/mRNA.

It was interesting to note that in the Pfizer "catchment" ie employee residential area, the fastest products to clear the shelves were: paper, disinfectant and...**ORGANIC TONIC WATER!!!**

I obtained the last pack of four!!!

In other words, in a residential area close to GSK and its affiliate Pfizer, *there was a run on tonic water, aka Hydroxyquinine...i.e., HCQ senza chlorine and sulphates.*

It is quite possible that its effectiveness in the treatment of "covid" or "vaccinoses" is due to its anti-coagulant properties, i.e., it melts the clots or impedes their formation.

Since writing this in 2020 I have encountered multiple persons forced to take the "covid" vax but surviving due to personal preferences for certain herbs, spices and tonics, all of which were anti-coagulant in nature.

What will Pfizer do now? Bribe Fauci's "replacement" in the NIH to announce hidden dangers in cinnamon and beer?

Nothing is beyond them; nothing is too ugly for the corrupt.

Peter McCullough: ...inflammation in the heart was coincident with the same pattern of inflammation in the arm. Thus we can conclude death within a few days of vaccination is most likely due to the genetic product and that inflammation in the arm may be a surrogate for a similar process in the heart. ..."

Well, d'uh! That's the immune system at work. Sending T4s and T8s to **identify** the "invader," histamines to fight it, accelerated blood flow to flush it out...

Only it doesn't "flush out."

T4s and T8s cannot identify the lab concocted and manufactured toxin, made by clueless "soyentists" with a lust for public funding, i.e., grant money, ie, living off the taxpayers while trying to *"depopulate" us!*

Which reveals the paucity of *natural intelligence* in academia today.

Because it would be *intelligent* to recognise that the remaining natural flora and fauna of the world have survived the same conditioning, meteorological changes, great and small, and other cycles affecting the world over centuries and have adapted accordingly with a subliminal resonance to other living entities.

Of course, there is nothing "natural" about the "soyentists" who spend their lives destroying God's creatures for profit.

How could they acknowledge that there is a connection between every living entity and then profiteer by its destruction! So "move God out...?"

Christians might call said connection a "Divine bond," but other faiths, religions and even primitives have also recognised super or preternatural influences, ie metaphysical energies resonating throughout the ages and consonant with Creation. Secularists prefer to say "nature," denying the existence of our Creator - which is interesting as the "soy-entists" or destroyers of "nature" have yet to create one single cell out of nothingness. Whereas ... "in the beginning..."[42]

To answer to the Creator requires following the Laws of Creation. To take down the shingle of faked "omnipotence" means sacrificing the adulation and profiteering afforded to dangerous persons such as Anthony Fauci and Bill Gates, along with their cohorts. But what doth it profit a man if he gains the whole world but loses his soul...

---

[42] The Holy Bible. Genesis.

What does that money and adulation mean when every day the fruits of your evil work are before you in the news, in the neighborhood, in the *Emergency Rooms? The Funeral Homes, the cemeteries...?*

Are the Fauci's, Gates and Schwabs, et al, so evil, so devoid of humanity that they perceive the suffering and deaths of their fake "vaccines" as triumphs? As evidence of their power to con humanity? To buy politicians? To corrupt the media and their colleagues in medicine and **pharm**a?

It would appear that they are not alone.

Silicon Valley is fully of techies joyfully anticipating the right to "chop off arms" and worse - in order to synthesise humanity into hybrid humanoid robots.

That Jeffrey Epstein was engaged in funding research into such lethal practices, along with a multitude of "high level" i.e., self-aggrandising associates suggests loudly and clearly that the motivation is not toward the benefit of humanity, but to create, wait for it, yet another Ho'wood "psy ops mind prep" image, the *minion...*

https://www.technology.org/2020/06/16/immortal-silicon-valley-top-transhumanist-projects-and-startups/

We've always had our Dr Frankensteins and Dr Crippens, Mengheles, Kevorkians, etc., but the mere idea of "silicon valley's"techies collaborating with Dr Fauci's "trained to kill" "soyentists" kind of chills the very marrow of one's bones...way beyond the "blood running cold."

After all we saw the product of the Fauci-Ghates collusion with "covid" and the rNA – DNA death jab.

So yes, an experiment in TRANSHUMANISM.

If you are still attached to pharma meds, but scared about the effects of the ModeRNA, Pfizer, Janssen and Janssen and Astra Zeneca, you might find this helpful.

If you're concerned about clot shots, do the opposite - unless you are a "bleeder" – in which case, read and follow closely.

Keep CHOCOLATE on standby, organic, dark, preferably. Or CHEESE, if Chocolate is unavailable.

If you are a "bleeder" or slow to clot, ***avoid*** alcohol, cinnamon, clover, quinine, etc.

https://www.wikihow.com/Make-Blood-Coagulate-Faster

There are remedies which I will not share publicly, because they require a level of expertise. They may be helpful in incising the fibrinogens and allowing for resorption – excretion of the fibrins or dissolution of the clots without use of heparin or other strong "blood thinners."

However, *they are not for use by amateurs. Especially amateurs with MD degrees, whose "substrate" is fundamentally antagonistic to the human immune system, and whose abuse of our remedies is often an abomination.*

*NO! The skilled, authentic Homeopath will find the most helpful remedies, choose the **one** that is correct for the presenting patient and **follow very carefully and closely, at each stage of recovery.***

The Homeopath treats *the patient,* not the ICD code!

Listing the "totality of symptoms"and reviewing carefully at each stage of recovery is essential.

One set of symptoms can be elided – not suppressed, eliminated, leading to revelation of causative factors or original symptoms, often suppressed by prescription meds.

There's an old saying among Homeopaths to the effect that "It takes ten years to make a Homeopath."

There's an element of truth in that. Even after thirty years, this profound system, "Gift of a Gracious God," continues to awe and surprise me.

Pharma has made it extremely difficult to practice according the essential, wise protocols of Hahnemann, but, according to the Gamaliel principle: "If it is from God it will survive."

Having a knowledge of the "oriental pulses," can also prove invaluable in assessing the *progress* of the chosen remedy along with observation of symptom status.

"Your voicemail is attached. Here is a transcription of the message content:

"Hi Dr. McNamara this is (former patient) calling and I just called to say thank you for all the good advice and remedies that you introduced me to and help me with a long life and know I'm doing pretty well right now and by the grace of God and I just wanted to say thank you to you. You've helped me and others even animals. So I just wanna wish you blessings and praise the Lord. Find out."

I had lost touch with that dear patient since first targeted by "harma."

22. STATS and FACTS

UK Surveys 1968, 1970:

A. 19.7% of allopaths' patients contracted flu! **Only 6/5%** of Homeopaths' patients contracted flu.
B. Number of **working days lost** by allopaths' patients was **six times** that of the Homeopaths!

Note, while our patients normally enjoy above average health and quality of life, most people consult a Homeopath as a last resort, when all else has failed and chronic ill health appears inevitable.

Mortality rate in allopathic hospitals was 33% higher than that in Homeopathic Hospitals – despite the worst cases being dumped on Homeopathic Hospitals.

NY Life Insurance companies gave Homeopaths' patients a 10% discount in recognition of faster recoveries, fewer complications.

In mid 19th century cholera epidemics, Homeopathy's survival rate was double or threefold that of the Allopaths:

1831, Austria: Allopathy's survival rate – 50%
                      Homeopathy's – 79.9 – 97.6

1849 Cincinnati: Allopathy – 40-52%
                      Homeopathy – 97%

1854 UK: Allopathy – 44%

                      Homeopathy – 84%

Spanish flu epidemic, 1917-1918.

Homeopathy's patients enjoyed a 97.6% survival rate.

Allopaths lost 35% of their patients, *over one third! Some even dumped their sickest patients into the Homeopathic Hospitals!*

Obviously Homeopathy was a threat to the **pharma** – petrochemical industry.

In the 1920s the pogroms started to close our schools and practices.

23. <u>**CVD 19 – LIES, DAMN LIES AND STATISTICS!**</u>

(Circa 2019)

Once upon a time, well after there "were wolves in Wales," and long after the "birds in red flannel petticoats" had flown the pond and become "cardinals" in the Colonies, there were "Cowboys and Indians."   Then political correctness gave us "good sheriffs" and "Bad Barts."

Because Bolsheviks flooded into the USA, disguised as poor, pathetic refugees, and took over the educational system, and the hearts and minds of our children and terrorized the authentic refugees from Soviet Communism.

Suddenly one plus one no longer equaled two, but a long series of words replaced numbers and confused our children. Computation became an exasperating narrative of anomalous, polysyllabic word strings. Deborah Birx is an outstanding example of its mind numbing effects as she clenches her fists, Pelosi-Clinton style, and reiterates misappropriated polysyllables such as "granulation" for charts and diagrams which show nothing of disease progression or human suffering. For me, she is forever associated with the term: "Lies, damned lies and statistics" Statistics useless for the care and treatment of the suffering, but essential for the tracking of the "failed" CV19, to ensure that CV 2020 blooms just in time for maximum damage on Nov 3, 2020.

Math is its own language: unique, direct and highly informative. It does not need an awkward and portentious patois. But we know that. Speaking French, English, German and Italian simultaneously or in rapid sequence might be fun for a while, but is not recommended as a method of instruction and results in gibberish.

"Gibberish" is derived from "gibbet" or apparatus from which humans were once hanged. A "flibberdigibbet" was an evil spirit who flew by the gibbets (scaffolds) seeking to capture the dying soul and take him/her to hell. Gibberish may be the language of the terrified, or the language of the dark side. Where Birx, Fauxci, Redfield and Hahn's "sound and fury signifying nothing" is concerned, the "dark side" seems to be the most likely source.

Unlike the UK where creativity and independent thought was encouraged, the NY Public School teachers found a way to make discovery and education an onerous, punitive, exercise in conditioning children to fill out forms and "just follow orders." This transformation was instigated by the Bolsheviks who infiltrated the USA disguised as "refugees." Does this sound familiar? Oh yes, there were authentic refugees…but allegedly the Obama sponsoring, Pritzkers were not in the patriot brigade, just committed Communist exports from the USSR.

Bad Bart suddenly became the "good guy," the victim, and the "Good Sheriff" was now the villain…how *dare* he love his country, his constitution, history, traditions, family and law and order! And shock, horror, dismay, the Good Sheriff carried a *gun!* Bad Bart's guns were ignored along with every incendiary item including words and ideology!

And so, when the Good Sheriff comes into town, takes out the bad guys, makes the streets safe for work, for leisure, for enterprise and brings it all back to life, and the people start to cheer, in comes Bad Bart, with a mask and a sneer.

The weak cower in fear – and blame the Good Sheriff.

And so, to show Bad Bart they're on his side, they wear a mask and sneer and jeer.

And plant their roadblocks everywhere.

The manner in which vents were used may[43] have caused more fatalities than the CV virus. Proning patients, sedating or paralyzing them puts them at risk of clots, and pushing pressurized oxygen into damaged lungs is insanity – unless the intent is death, in which case it is homicidal. "Antagonistic" medicine has other resources which have not even been considered!

The speed at which NY Hospitals ran out of paralysands cries out for Federal Investigation.

The absence of official autopsies, likewise.

The "set dressing" of trucks outside Elmhurst and other City Hospitals, likewise.

Likewise, the skewed logistics regarding "co-morbidities" and extreme mortality rate among the elderly.

Yes, I am asking for a serious and intense inquiry into the likelihood that Senior Citizens were murdered in NY Hospitals, subsequent to the removal of their organs. It appears likely that, under the transplanted, wannabe transgender, Dr Richard aka Rachel Levine, this also occurred in PA. Dr. Levine transferred hospitalised patients, with an allegedly highly contagious virus, into Nursing Homes, while putting his own mother into a private hotel.

---

[43] It is now well established that the proning and the high pressure venting on Remdesivir damaged lungs were the primary cause of "covid" deaths.

Yes, the mortality rate soared in PA too. Governor Tom Wolfe is now replaced – by his former Attorney General who tacitly colluded in the unlawful deaths of thousands of Pennsylvanians. Investments in Pfizer?

Paralysands are used in the removal of organs from living patients, a common practice in China, and reportedly in the USA.

Did Fauci bring this criminal practice from China to the USA?

PA's former Sec of Health is a man who pretends he is a woman. Whether he believes it or is hiding from litigation relevant to previous employment as a psychiatrist working with vulnerable teenagers is relevant to the mental health and motivation of [44]Richard aka Rachel Levine, now an "unadmirable" admiral in the US Navy...reward for bad behavior?

Added to that, his experience is primarily in New York City. I have considerable experience with the corruption and evil of NYC and NYS' corruption and venality toward the dying. Richard aka Rachel Levine, the shrink with the ongoing identity crisis who controls PA's Health Services needs to be accountable. In compromising the health and lives of PA's Seniors, Levine's actions are questionably consistent with those of the dying State of NY, a State executed by its own Governor.

And still the slaughter continues...

---

[44] Moderna CEO Stephane Bancel admits company made 100K COVID-19 vaccine doses in 2019 before the pandemic even started (newstarget.com)

FIRST. DO. NO. HARM.[45]

---

45 First line of the Hippocratic Oath.

24. PRIVATE NOTES MADE PUBLIC

In light of the ongoing lies and perjuries © **D.McNamara**

1. Vitamin B 12 injectible is available over the counter in many developed countries.
2. It is not available in the USA without a prescription and a bureaucratic "fandango." [46]
3. It is happily prescribed for persons with sickle cell anemia, for which it is helpful but *not specific.*
4. It is specific for **pernicious anemia.**
5. **Pernicious anemia primarily affects persons of Scandinavian, Irish, English - the Vikings got around- or North European origin.**
6. **It is extremely difficult for a person of European ethnicity to obtain a prescription for B12 injectible in the USA, let alone obtain emergency use vials.**
7. **It is extremely difficult for a person of European ethnicity to obtain a *diagnosis* of Pernicious Anemia.**
8. **Although symptoms were perfectly obvious to the author at the age of 11, they were ignored by her GP who went on to be the Dean of one of the more prestigious Medical Schools in Europe, even as his patient/s deteriorated. This arrogance or ignorance, deliberate or**

---

1. [46] (Complex Latin American Dance.)

otherwise is inexcusable, pervasive and permeates P*harma medicine.

9. Symptoms attributed to the MTHFR Gene are identical to those persons with correct diagnoses of pernicious anemia.

10. Symptoms attributed to Alzheimers and Parkinsons are identical to persons with correct diagnoses of pernicious anemia.

11. Persons suffering with undiagnosed pernicious anemia are most likely to be diagnosed with anything but the blatantly obvious.

12. That B12 is used adjunctively for sickle cell, and that black babies are routinely tested for sickle cell anemia, and that B12 injectible is used for domestic pets and live-stock but is **highly restricted from white European Americans** *crosses the line into racist genocide in the Medico-pHARMaceutical professions, headed, most notoriously by Fauci, Gates, Redfield, Bourla etc.*

13. *It could simply be that white European Americans are perceived as enjoying "good health insurance..."* therefore easy targets for long, protracted and costly health "care." Or, something even more sinister, given that 88% of the targeted transgender children are white, middle class.

Please note the following: The misdiagnosed conditions listed affected mostly Scandinavians and white persons of Northern European heritage, and in the US, i.e., persons of mid to high income in areas dominated by the pharmaceutical industry.

Note also, that at an age when B12 absorption diminishes, the Medical cartels advise "low cholesterol diets." Which translate as limited beef, liver, eggs, etc.

In other words: LIMITED, RESTRICTED B12 leads to DEPRIVATION of a substance vital for the development of healthy red blood cells, ie oxygen carriers and for the development and maintenance of the vulnerable CENTRAL NERVOUS SYSTEM!

The long term effects of B12 Deprivation are IDENTICAL TO:

ALZHEIMERS!
PARKINSONS!
AMNESIA!
DYSNOMIA!

Can be "induced" by prolonged adherence to vegetarian and vegan diets, but *primarily affects persons of Scandinavian or North European heritage.*

Such persons, by dint of hard work and foresight managed to acquire property and lands, now greatly coveted.

ARE YOU THERE YET?

GENOCIDE?

25. CANCER – A CONTRARY OPINION

In my observation and work with the Human Immune System, it has become clear that the "economy" of the body is paramount

The vital organs are the priority: the brain, the lungs, liver, etc., all essential to survival.

When there is a toxic overload, and for reasons internal or external, the organs of digestion, elimination, the liver, kidney, spleen, rbcs, wbcs, leukocytes, lymphocytes, T4s, T8s, etc., cannot resolve or dissolve, or eliminate toxins, albeit organic or inorganic, they are stored in the liver to be released at the first sign of homeostasis - or metabolic stability. That would be, say, a period of adequate rest, accompanied by a healthy diet and minimum stress. The release of such toxins, e.g., in the case of an alcoholic gives rise, thence, to the "phenomenon" of the "dry drunk...."

This occurs when, after prolonged abstention, a person afflicted with the alcoholic syndrome starts to enjoy a restoration to good health, aka "recovery." When the immune system recognizes a level of "homeostasis" or metabolic equilibrium, the liver starts to release quantities of alcohol stored there, in the interest of the survival of the person concerned. This gives the appearance of inebriation and the heroic recovering alcoholic is too often suspected of returning to old habits.

While the periodic release of stored toxins inevitably extends the life of the person concerned, it can be disconcerting and even distressing.

Where inorganic, genetically inappropriate "materials" ie alien cells and tissue are concerned, the response is not so simple.

With the unconscionable, increased contamination of the human genome with cells from canines, murdered prenatal infants, rodents, simians, etc., in the so called "vaccination" system, said contaminants are "poured" into the bodies of infants, whose meiosis and mitosis – cell division and replication and development occur at a rapid rate.

Inserting the mitochondria or DNA/RNA or any live genetic material to the body of an infant is evil.

"First Do No Harm" and the rest of the Hippocratic Oath were discarded in 1973 coincident with the passage of Roe v Wade allowing medical personnel to perform abortion, an act that was considered abhorrent for centuries.

Mitochondria, energy producing "entity" within cells create proteins that manufacture the energy necessary for metabolism. Rather than go down the rabbit hole of tons of incidental data, I'll just postulate that the mitochondrial "crista" or core contains AMP,[47] one of the components of the host's RNA, and also controls or organises the other phosphate nucleotides.

These all play vital parts in the synthesis of respiration, the protection of cells, and host or "native" RNA, and the production of riboproteins.

---

[47] AMP: Adenosine monophosphate; ADP: Adenosine diphosphate and ATP: Adenosine triphosphate.

The introduction of alien RNA into the Human mitochondria, or attempts thereto will result in a synthesized attack protein, and the metabolic destruction of the alien RNA.

If, however, the introduction is via a vial of multiple toxins and biohazards such as the rodent or macaque monkey RNA in ModeRNA, the result is chaos and confusion. To which threat will the bacterial monitoring ribosomes respond?

This confusion within the "cellular intelligence" as we Homeopaths would otherwise, simply put it, buys time allows the mitoribosome or riboprotein to *begin* "integrating," or "translating" alien mRNA...until the "cytokine" storm dies down, ie, the normal responses to bacterial invasion, eg, fever, sweating, epistaxis, rhinitis, coughs, etc., die down.

The bioweapon aka "vaccine" is the biochemical equivalent of the Trojan Horse. A surprise attack on the immune system.

T4 and T8 cells are "miraculous" when it comes to identifying and destroying *biochemical pathogens;* do they have the "sophistication" to identify alien RNA?

Perhaps not.

And perhaps that's what bought the invaders "time..." Time for at least a partial integration or "knitting" of alien RNA with the host or human RNA, resulting in the lethal fibrinogens, formerly referred to as "clots."

These would be teratogens...mini monsters, sneaking into the human biome, growing within it while the immune system initially attacked other pathogens in the deadly shots.

But the mitochondria AMP eventually said, "No, we can't and won't work with this. Begone."

Thus, the complex systems of defense described in previous chapters, then unwittingly, become the killers.

Diabolical. To use the Creator's brilliant protective systems against His beloved people.

"Pharmakopeia." Just another word for sorcery.

The following is creepy, but it does address the ethos and attitudes of many supporters and associates of Fauci, Ghates, et al, and the extreme amorality of the Pharmaceutical industries associated with the development of the lethal "vaccines."

https://rumble.com/v1mej10-a-demon-spills-the-beans-about-covid-jabs-sudden-death-and-the-soul.html

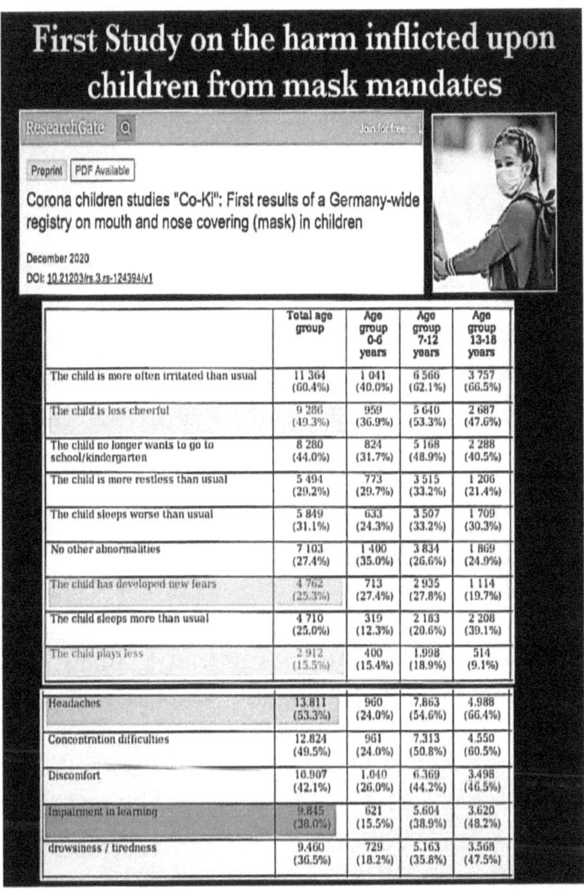

First Study on the harm inflicted upon children from mask mandates

Preprint | PDF Available

Corona children studies "Co-Ki": First results of a Germany-wide registry on mouth and nose covering (mask) in children

December 2020

DOI: 10.21203/rs.3.rs-124394/v1

	Total age group	Age group 0-6 years	Age group 7-12 years	Age group 13-18 years
The child is more often irritated than usual	11 364 (60.4%)	1 041 (40.0%)	6 566 (62.1%)	3 757 (66.5%)
The child is less cheerful	9 286 (49.3%)	959 (36.9%)	5 640 (53.3%)	2 687 (47.6%)
The child no longer wants to go to school/kindergarten	8 280 (44.0%)	824 (31.7%)	5 168 (48.9%)	2 288 (40.5%)
The child is more restless than usual	5 494 (29.2%)	773 (29.7%)	3 515 (33.2%)	1 206 (21.4%)
The child sleeps worse than usual	5 849 (31.1%)	633 (24.3%)	3 507 (33.2%)	1 709 (30.3%)
No other abnormalities	7 103 (27.4%)	1 400 (35.0%)	3 834 (26.6%)	1 869 (24.9%)
The child has developed new fears	4 762 (25.3%)	713 (27.4%)	2 935 (27.8%)	1 114 (19.7%)
The child sleeps more than usual	4 710 (25.0%)	319 (12.3%)	2 183 (20.6%)	2 208 (39.1%)
The child plays less	2 912 (15.5%)	400 (15.4%)	1.998 (18.9%)	514 (9.1%)
Headaches	13.811 (53.3%)	960 (24.0%)	7.863 (54.6%)	4.988 (66.4%)
Concentration difficulties	12.824 (49.5%)	961 (24.0%)	7.313 (50.8%)	4.550 (60.5%)
Discomfort	10.907 (42.1%)	1.040 (26.0%)	6.369 (44.2%)	3.498 (46.5%)
Impairment in learning	9.845 (38.0%)	621 (15.5%)	5.604 (38.9%)	3.620 (48.2%)
drowsiness / tiredness	9.460 (36.5%)	729 (18.2%)	5.163 (35.8%)	3.568 (47.5%)

Where were the educators? The science teachers, the biology professors?

Where were the projects, the investigations, the examination of masks under school microscopes?

Where the simple experiments?

Not even considered!

And then came the lockdowns, presumably to avoid such projects or the possibility thereof among other motivations!

26. RECAP

Since I started writing "Protocols" (working title) torrents of information, factual reports, data, is appearing daily in both social media, Main Stream Media, and Official "Government" Agencies. In addition to which, a tsunami of professional witnesses have also come forward to testify against the lethal GMO bio-hazard aka the "Covid" "vaccine," or more colloquially, the "clotshot" or "deathjab."

I cannot provide direct links to *all* professional studies, for this reason:

The NIH lied – to me – claiming that I "mass" down load papers in their Pub Med Files.

For the record, this is false. Downloading papers from NIH Pub med Files is a rare event for me. The last thing I want to or need to read are NIH's cluttered and derivative "peer reviewed" files.

How on earth did "peer review" get to be a "good thing" in a climate of ferocious and amoral agenda-driven academic competition, bribery and corruption, plagiary and theft.

I can only speculate as to if or how many helpful discoveries by emergent scientists were either stolen or buried by the chiefs at NIH, NAIAD, CDC, FDA, etc.

And if you question my cynicism, I have two words: Dr Fauci. Would any student or young researcher have the courage – or professional "stupidity" to challenge the sources of Fauci's abundant patents?   So many of America's "prominent" "geniuses" have been **proven** plagiarists, but continue to profit from their stolen intellectual properties. The sheer number of patents registered to that equivocating "soy-entist,'" ie, Anthony Fauci, combined with the complete absence of intelligence in the design of the death jab makes the provenance of said patents suspect – unless the "vaccine" was *intended* for use as a weapon of mass destruction, i.e., depopulation or genocide.

If I download any NIH files it is to prove and corroborate any statements that I may make in my own analyses of this horrendous "scamdemic" and promotion of a deadly genetic bioweapon, **or, most disturbing to them, to challenge decisions or premises on which certain decisions are made**.

So, if you are interested in Truth, Justice, and the survival of the Human Race, then I invite you to make your own journey through the morass of lies, disinformation, cruelty, medical murder, media involvement, political machinations and compromise and the grief and sorrow of millions of people around the world that is the official "Covid" and "clotshot" narrative.

From Genghis Khan to Attila the Hun, through Napoleon, Stalin, Lenin, Marx, Hitler, there have been men – and some women – willing to destroy their brothers and sisters on planet earth...

For money, for power, for land, or from what the Homeopaths would call a "syphilitic diathesis," cruelty and sadism being the outcome of the second and third stages of that dreaded disease.

The Tudors certainly stand as examples of that, Henry VIII degrading from a sensitive musician to a sadistic and cruel murderer due to the degradation of cerebral nerves and tissue.

His daughter, Elizabeth 1, was born with his syphilis, and wore lead based make up to cover the pox marks. Her half-sister, "Bloody Mary," also appears to have inherited the syphilitic diathesis from her father, Henry VIII and the sterility that accompanied it, leading to suspicions of witchcraft, the village abortionists being designated "witches."

For this reason Elizabeth I declined to marry taking on the rubric of the "Virgin Queen..."

A clever but evil substitution for the now forbidden "Virgin Mary," whose image her soldiers destroyed at every opportunity.

And that pox which so embarrassed the savage Queen became the focus of the cruel and sadistic experiments in "vaccination" by which Dr Edward Jenner sought to prevent and cure it.

He seemed to have heard one of the principles of Homeopathy, that is, "similia similibus curenter," id est, "let like cure like..." but he didn't get the rest of it.

He saw cowpox on the hands of a milkmaid and its similarity to the pustules of smallpox and made a crude decoction.

He tried it on his own son, killed him and then a number of his neighbours and wanted to stop, but Big Pharma took over and the rest is history. Vaccines became a "license to kill..."

That is: "THE SINS OF THE FATHERS ARE VISITED ON THEIR CHILDREN?

Interesting how ambitious ghouls use their own children as guinea pigs.

What hope, then, for the survival of any stranger who falls into their clutches.[48]

The first flu epidemic followed the first attempt to mass vaccinate with the "flu virus.

Ironically, Semmelweiss and Pasteur, like Jenner, were inspired by Samuel Hahnemann.

None of them, however, actually understood the power and precision of Homeopathy although Semmelweiss took Hahnemann's "peripheral" admonitions to heart and started washing his hands after delivering babies, instead of wiping them on a blood encrusted jacket, like Fauci's soul mates of the 18th century.

The filthier the jacket, the more esteemed the surgeon/ obstetrician. They would strut the streets in their filthy jackets, arrogant to the hilt, despite the death toll of

---

[48] There are dedicated allopaths who put their patients welfare above income, status, bribes, "symposia," ie free vacays, status boosters, etc. I've had the privilege of working with them, for the benefit of the patient, but I would not "out" them. Two whom I praised publicly retired soon after, etc., etc. Coincidentally, of course! Sad when the so called "healing" industry acts more like an organised crime syndicate!

thousands of babies and new mothers dying from the puerperal fever spread from doctor to patient to infant by their arrogance and ignorance of basic hygiene.

Something akin to Fauci's death toll, because puerperal fever was an epidemic *caused* by the "esteemed soy-entists" of the day. Flu epidemic, likewise! Flu season follows *Flu vax season!*

Pasteur took "asepsis," i.e., cleanliness, to another level, i.e., anti-sepsis and the pasteurisation of milk, still controversial.

It was, Jenner, however, who would become Fauci's "exemplar" Would Fauci be arrogant and ambitious enough to vaccinate his son – if he had one?

He will go down as one of the most infamous characters in history. Fauci and Gates – sociopath and psychopath? One enjoys the power but is indifferent to the suffering. The other really, really enjoys all the suffering that he can afflict: all the deaths, the fatalities, mortalities, conjoin to feed the "God" complex.

The remark: "when men try to be angels, they become as monsters," is attributed to French philosopher Blaise Pascal.

To which I add, "when men appoint themselves as "deities" they become as devils," evil incarnate and below any human level of stupidity and ignorance.

They "know" everything but understand **nothing!**

The problem is, the public believes billion dollar media campaigns, which involve funding soap operas and prime time TV shows all glorifying p*harm*a meds and always finding a way to denigrate Homeopathy in one form or the other. Usually with a completely fabricated story line, sometimes with just a comment.

I expect that from American TV, but was surprised to see it in "Doc Martin," i.e., Martin Clunes, the actor, last seen ogling me over a breakfast room at a nice hotel in Ireland, where he was taking part in a shoot of farmed pheasant. All the joys of shooting a pheasant that has no place to hide.

Something akin to Pfizer's researchers tossing live rats into their grinders and laughing at their agony.[49]

Hmmm. I would have kept Martin's "shady" pheasant shoot to myself if it were not for the "one liner" in "Doc Martin" denigrating Homeopathy!

I would like to know if he was paid extra for that filth.

Free Speech is no excuse for keeping the public ignorant of the suffering Homeopathy uniquely relieves, even as their children and other loved ones die from conditions resolvable and curable by skilled, authentic Homeopaths.

And those who are paying optimum premiums for "good medical insurance," might consider those premiums would plummet as the efficacy of Homeopathy also provides significant cost savings to

---

[49] Eye witness. Protected source.

the Insurance Providers. So much so, that they once offered Homeopathy's patients significant discounts!

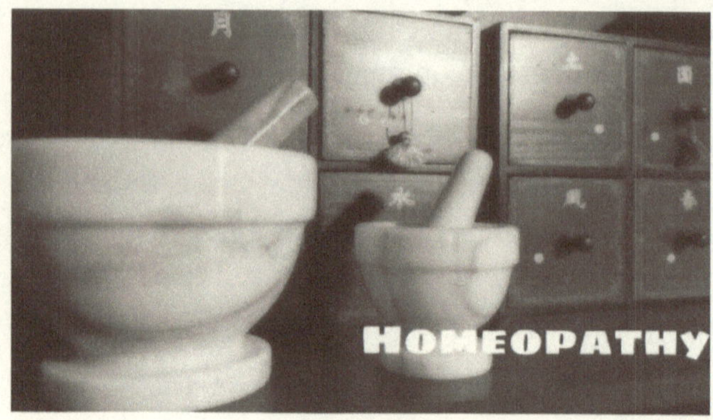

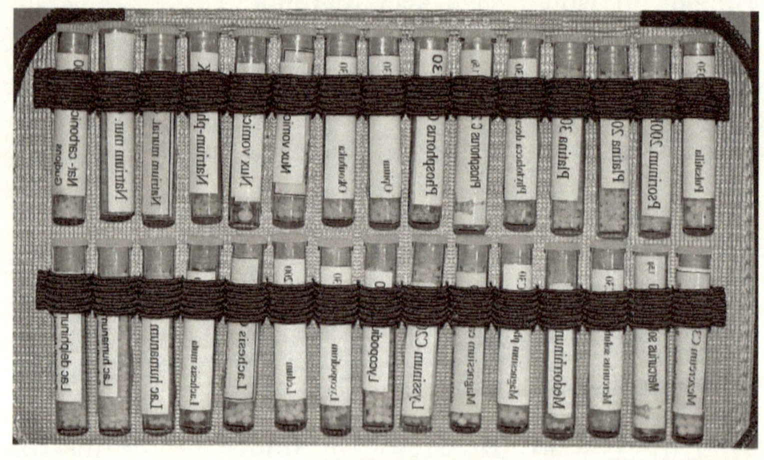

Just a small portion of the authentic Homeopath's "arsenal"

Deirdre McNamara, D.Hom made History by being the first Homeopath to consult in an NY Hospital in over a century.

Prior to two attempts on her life by Cuomo's NYS thugs, her work weaned long term (16 months) patients off respirators, curing anti biotic resistant infections, and restoring motion and sensation to paralysed limbs.

*Saving to the State of NY was about $1,000,000 per annum, **per patient**, with joyful results to said patients.*

Dr D received the personal and written thanks of the late (St) Mother Teresa for her Homeopathic work. St Mother Teresa now has Homeopathic clinics all over Calcutta.

As an author, McNamara's "Tribe of Cannibals: Operation Take Down America" reveals a subversive arrangement between Columbia U, George Soros, Obama and Holder to destroy Constitutional America – a 40 year experiment that failed and cost the US Taxpayer dearly.

She has a 100% survival and rapid recovery rate in patients presenting with confirmed diagnoses of "Covid 19."

Other successes include: Immediate relief and full recovery within one week of patient suffering recurrent episodes of MRSA. Same patient on respirator for 16 months. Within a month of treatment, patient breathing room air, etc.

Complete cures and negative viral load in patients presenting with confirmed diagnoses of Hepatitis A, B, C.

Stopped vax related seizures in three year old child in UK. Almost immediately. Last report no further seizures.

Accelerated symphysis of fracture (humerus) in octagenarian patient with osteoporosis.

Accelerated symphysis of fracture (tallus) in Senior Citizen. Rapidity of recovery alarmed orthopedist!

Restored sensation and movement in both post thrombosis paralysis and post traumatic paralysis.

Correctly diagnosed and cured cholecystitis where NY Hospital failed on both counts.

Prevented complete and permanent loss of sight in young man in substance abuse recovery center; symptoms missed or ignored by attending physician. Glaucoma confirmed by opthalmologist.

*Correctly diagnosed porphyria and suspected cerebro-spinal tumor in the family of a TCD Dean of Medicine,oblivious to the symptoms. Homeopath **not** invited to consult on treatment. Both patients died, most likely of radiation poisoning. TCD is a prestigious European University*

Her dramas were performed to SRO audiences in NY, and her published books include: "Homeopathy in the Time of Covid," "Tribe of Cannibals: Operation Take Down America," "Heart of Mercy," "The Sanity of Christ vs the Fallacies of Freud," "A Whisper of Angels," "The Tuscany Express" (Homeopathy in Travel Emergencies) "Child Sexual Abuse: Never Call it Love," "SOS – For Survivors of Suicides," "New Christmas Stories for Children of All

Ages," "Christmas – The Gracious Time," and many others.

She also composes liturgical music; works performed in NY and NJ.

Works written prior to 2001 are archived in the National Library of Ireland, and the U.S. Library of Congress.

She has many awards and citations to her credit and is the daughter of scientist and publisher Derry and artist Phyllis Kelleher, and grand-daughter of (Sir) Charles Kellman, explorer and broadcaster and Gwendoline Kellman.

Dr Kelleher-McNamara was born in Trinidad, WI while her father was a scientist employed by British Food Research, and returned to England at the age of ten months. She was considered a prodigy, tests showing the literary equivalency of an Oxbridge grad at the age of nine as well as accelerated in Math, Science and Music.

After moving to Ireland she won many awards and citations despite physical frailty. At the age of 11 she correctly diagnosed the cause of her fragile health, but was ignored by the "Deans of Medicine" there and in the USA.

Homeopathy transformed her health – a Gift to be shared.

Since I started putting "Potentials" in book form, there has been a tsunami of supportive testimonies, evidence, lab reports, articles, videos, social media outrage, litigation, etc., upholding and proving the validity of my words and concerns *ab initio*.

"Protocols" barely touches the surface of the depravity and evil behind the masks, lockdowns, lethal jabs etc. There is little to support the contention that "covid" was a "public health" issue. It has the hallmark of a private financial strategy and issue!

However, the media still continues to hide the truth and collude with evil. Genocide is evil. Bravo to the great people now standing against it.

For that reason I refrain from expressing my gratitude to the great people of America, Ireland, N. Ireland, England, Italy, Spain, Canada, Australia who stood by me through three challenging years.

Christians of the world unite; you have everything to lose: your lives, your families, your great music, art authentic science and architecture, your health, your education and judicial systems and your Right to practice your Faith.

"Be not afraid. I go before you always." Christo Rex.

ADDENDUM: MULTI SOURCE TESTIMONIES

The bioweapon – falsely termed a "vaccine" and falsely advertised as protection against a falsified "pandemic" has caused untold suffering, pain, disfigurement, disability and death to millions of innocent citizens around the world.

They and their loved ones deserve to be heard, so I am including some of the voices here below. As far as I know they are in the public domain but I will gladly elide if requested by the citizen testifying.

*One of the first to stand up was Nichole Belland, **pharmacy manager** for Safeway store at 1892 of Cortez in Lacey-Olympia Safeway: "I quit effective immediately because I will not give this poison to people. Wake up, everybody. This is poison. This is hurting people. I've seen it. I've seen customers die. Wake up, do not take it." – Nichole Belland, 2020.*

In a sane world she would receive a Congressional Medal of Honor. I salute her!

Incentivized to Kill: Government Bounties on American Lives

"Hospitals get paid an enormous amount if they use Remdesivir," informed Dr. Peterson Pierre. "20% surcharge on the entire hospital bill."

"They also get paid extra if they use a ventilator, and they get paid extra for COVID deaths. So for each patient, you're looking at about a $400,000 to $500,000 bounty."

Source (https://rumble.com/v1z842v-daily-dose-why-doctors-are...)Follow @VigilantFox

Rumble (https://rumble.com/v1zunuk-incentivized-to-kill...) | Substack (http://thevigilantfox.substack.com/) | Support (https://www.redvoicemedia.com/vigilantfox/) | Socials (https://bio.site/vigilantfox)

So DEATH *was* the objective. Mass Murder.

"Depopulation" sounds far more civilized than **GENOCIDE!**

At least to the criminally insane!

Points of Interest:

https://knowledgeburrow.com › how-long-does-it-take-for-blood-to-coagulate-on-the-floor

How long does it take for blood to coagulate on the floor?

Jan 23, 2021**How long** does it take for **blood to coagulate** after a cut? Monitor the length of time that a minor cut bleeds. The most telling sign that your **blood** is not coagulating fast enough is excessive bleeding. It should not take longer than ten minutes for a small cut or scrape to stop bleeding, with anywhere from one to nine minutes being normal.

https://www.quora.com › How-long-does-it-take-for-blood-to-coagulate-1?share=1

How long does it take for blood to coagulate? - Quora

In vitro, a properly collected tube of unanticoagulated whole **blood** collected in a tube with no additive should fully clot within 30 minutes. This is provided the patient isn't on a **blood** thinner and the **blood** wasn't drawn from a heparin lock. Different tube types cause **blood to coagulate** at different rates.

https://www.wikihow.com › Make-Blood-Coagulate-Faster

3 Ways to Make Blood Coagulate Faster - wikiHow

Dec 27, 2021It should not take longer than ten minutes for a small cut or scrape to stop bleeding, with anywhere from one to nine minutes being normal. If you are still bleeding after ten minutes, see a doctor as soon as possible. [5] If you or someone else is losing substantial amounts of **blood**, provide first aid and get to a hospital as quickly as possible.

https://www.healthline.com › health › coagulation-tests

Coagulation Tests: Types, Procedure, and Results - Healthline

It normally takes about 25 to 30 seconds. It may take longer if you take **blood** thinners. Other reasons for abnormal results include hemophilia, liver disease, and malabsorption. It's also useful...

https://healthfully.com › long-blood-circulate-5397064.html

How Long Does It Take Blood to Circulate? | Healthfully

The **blood** vessels in a child's body would be more than 60,000 miles **long**. **Blood** takes less time to circulate when you are active or exercising, as your heart rate decreases when you are resting 1.

G woundcaresociety.org › long-long-cut-bleed

How long is too long for a cut to bleed - Wound Care Society

You should seek medical attention if your cut bleeds for more than 15 minutes after you put sufficient pressure. However, if you are under certain circumstances which affect the way your **blood coagulates**, you should not wait for 15 minutes once you have your skin cut. Otherwise, directly seek for medical attention and explain your conditions.

https://www.vikschaatcorner.com › how-long-does-it-take-for-blood-to-coagulate-after-death

How long does it take for blood to coagulate after death?

3-5 days after death — the body starts to bloat and **blood**-containing foam leaks from the mouth and nose. 8-10 days after death — the body turns from green to red as the **blood** decomposes and the organs in the abdomen accumulate gas. Several weeks after death — nails and teeth fall out. What happens to the body 36 hours after death?

https://citizens.news/688221.html

https://childrenshealthdefense.org/defender/fda-limits-j-j-vaccine-blood-clotting-disorder/?utm_source=salsa&eType=EmailBlastContent&eId=db437bc2-b0c0-457f-883e-19f43e55adf1

https://www.drugs.com › mtm › quinine.html

Quinine Uses, Side Effects & Warnings - Drugs.com

Mar 25, 2022 **Quinine** may cause serious side effects. Call your doctor at once if you have: fever, chills, body aches, flu symptoms, sores in your mouth and throat; easy bruising, unusual bleeding (nose, mouth, vagina, or rectum), purple or red pinpoint spots under your skin; headache with chest pain and severe dizziness, fainting, fast or pounding heartbeats;

And yet, in the supermarkets near Pfizer-GSK, organic quinine "tea" ie **tonic water,** sold out as rapidly as disinfectant and cleaning papers in the first days of the plandemic.

🌿https://www.pdsa.org › treatments › complementary › food-as-a-cure.html

<u>Platelet Disorder Support Association - for People with ITP - Eating ...</u>

Foods that can interfere with blood **clotting** Blueberries, red/purple grape products, garlic, onions, ginger, ginseng, and tomatoes have all been shown to prevent blood **clotting**. **Quinine** Avoid food and drinks containing **quinine**, including tonic water and bitter lemon and drinks; these can lower platelets. Don't Forget...

So, frankly, all of the foods listed above should be extremely helpful for all who took the "clot shot" whether wilfully, or by coercion or "jab or job" blackmail.

The following links lead to extensive research and detail on the background and development of the scamdemic and the genuine epidemic of GMO vaccinosis which followed as people panicked and allowed "trusted" health professionals to stick animal RNA into their arms and those of their children.

https://sashalatypova.substack.com/p/the-role-of-the-us-dod-and-their

https://boriquagato.substack.com/p/israeli-government-lost-the-agreement

https://www.westernjournal.com/lifestyle/

https://sashalatypova.substack.com/p/the-ballistics-report-is-in-pfizer

A really scary one: https://medicine.iu.edu/faculty-labs/corson/protocols/rna-precautions

https://rumble.com/v2ip9c0-shocking-testimony-from-two-canadian-funeral-industry-professionals.html

https://www.studysmarter.us/explanations/biology/energy-transfers/oxidative-phosphorylation/

...and so many more...

COURAGEOUS PROFESSIONAL WITNESSES TO VAX REACTIONS AND ER

Warning, there are going to be TRIGGERS throughout this. Skip this whole comment if sensitive.(DM)

As an E.R. nurse, I have seen the cover up. Where do you think kids go when they have a vaccine reaction? They go to the E.R. They come to me. I cannot even begin to guess how many times over the years I have seen vaccine reactions come through my E.R. Without any exaggeration, it has to be counted in hundreds. Sometimes it seemed like it was one or two cases in a single shift, every shift, for weeks. Then I would get a lull, and I wouldn't catch one for a week or two, then I'd catch another case per night for a couple weeks. This was common.

Once, I was training a nursing student, about to graduate, on their E.R. experience rotation in nursing school. This student and I floated up to triage to cover the triage nurse for a break. I was quizzing them on what to ask and look for as a triage nurse on pediatric kids that came through. I made a point about asking about immunizations right out the gates. The student was puzzled, and asked why, and I told the student because we see vaccine reactions every day and it is their job to catch it, alert the doctor and the parents, and report it to VAERS. Some higher power apparently smiled on my attempt to open the eyes of another nurse I guess, because not even ten minutes later, a woman brought her child up to the counter. Sudden onset super high fever and lethargy. I asked if the child was up to date on vaccination. The mother replied he had them just a few hours ago. I glanced at the student, who looked shocked and looked back at me in disbelief. I nodded, told them to remember this, and then took the mom and her child to finish the triage in back. When I was done I came back and sat down with the student, and asked what he learned that night so far. The first response: "What I was told about vaccines wasn't true". I couldn't have said it better. That student is going to go on to be like me, advocating for his patients with his eyes wide open.

The cases almost always presented similarly, and often no one else connected it. The child comes in with either a fever approaching 105F, or seizures, or lethargy or can't wake up, or sudden overwhelming sickness, screaming that won't stop, spasms, GI inclusion, etc.

And one of the first questions I would ask as triage nurse, was: are they current on their vaccinations? It's a safe question that nobody sees coming, and nobody understands the true impact of. Parents (and co-workers) usually just think I'm trying to rule out the vaccine preventable diseases, when in fact, I am looking to see how recently they were vaccinated to determine if this is a vaccine reaction. Too often I heard a parent say something akin to "Yes they are current, the pediatrician caught up their vaccines this morning during their check up, and the pediatrician said they were in perfect health!" If I had a dollar for every time I'd heard that, I could fly to Europe for free.

But here's the more disturbing part. For all the cases I've seen, I have NEVER seen any medical provider report them to VAERS. I have filed VAERS reports. But I am the ONLY nurse I have EVER met that files VAERS reports. I also have NEVER met a doctor that filed a VAERS report. Mind you, I have served in multiple hospitals across multiple states, alongside probably well over a hundred doctors and probably 300-400+ nurses. I've worked in big hospitals (San Francisco Bay Area Metro 40 bed ER, Las Vegas NV Metro 44 bed ER) and small hospitals (Rural access 2 bed ER, remote community 4 bed ER) and everything in between. When I say NEVER, I mean NEVER. I have even made a point of sitting in the most prominent spot at the nurses station filling out a VAERS report to make sure as many people saw me doing it as possible to generate the expected "what are you doing" responses to get that dialog going with people. And in every case, if a nurse approached me, their response was "I've never done that" or "I didn't know we could do that" or, worse "What is VAERS?" which was actually the most common response. The response from doctors? Silence. Absolute total refusal to engage in discussion or to even acknowledge what I was doing or what VAERS was.

The big take away from that? **VAERS is woefully underreported.** I am PROOF of that. The number one place parents bring their kids in the event of a vaccine reaction is the E.R., and as an E.R. staffer, I have NEVER met anyone who filed one, in spite of seeing hundreds of cases of obvious vaccine associated harm come through. What does that say about reported numbers? **The CDC/HHS admits that VAERS is under-reported, and probably only representative of 1/10th the actual number of injuries**. I contest that, and from personal experience, **I would say the numbers in VAERS are more like 1/1000th the actual numbers, not 1/10th.**

And the final part of that, is that I have, first hand, seen blatant cover ups from doctors. I have seen falsification of medical records and documentation via intentional omission. I have challenged doctors who refused to put in the chart that the child was vaccinated 4 hours ago and was in perfect health, and now suddenly they are non-responsive, seizing, febrile at 105, and that labs, LP, and imaging confirms cerebral edema /encephalitis. I reminded the doctor as they are writing their report that the child was vaccinated mere hours before. And at the end, there is total omission of this fact, and the physician pass-off notes state encephalitis of unknown origin. I ask the doctor if they will file a VAERS report, and they argue that this has nothing to do with it, as it is purely coincidental, and nothing should be filed; they are 'safe and effective.' I remind them that VAERS is a reporting body for ANY symptoms that are contemporaneous to vaccination, whether causation is believed to be associated or not, and I get the dismissal that they are not filing it because it has nothing to do with it.

No one brings it up to the parents.

It is this giant rug-sweep that happens, and any mention of the vaccination is systematically removed or withheld from the record. A perfect example of this, was an ambulance crew that came in with a pass-off report that included the fact the child had been vaccinated only hours prior to onset of symptoms. The physician made sure this pass-off sheet disappeared mysteriously and could not get filed with the patient medical record. So yes, I have seen the vaccine damage cover up first hand. I know that it is intentional and active in the medical community. I know that it is happening. And on top of total denial of any association, and total cover up, they also refuse to report to VAERS which is supposed to be reported to for ANYTHING that is even in NO WAY SUSPECTED to be associated with the vaccine. This is a systemic suppression of information and statistics.

And yes, in the cases described above, I did approach the parents, and I did tell them about

VAERS, and I did start a case for them and file a report. I did force the issue through my charting, although it will most likely be buried and overlooked.

I have experienced the corruption and suppression of the truth in the medical community about vaccines first hand from the provider perspective. It does happen. Every day.

To catch the entire thread (long but I highly recommend it, especially if you're into reading and analyzing studies.

http://community.babycenter.com/.../pretty_simple_explanation...

The original post was made on page 12 in the link above, if anyone wants to copy and share.

Meanwhile, back at the White House in 2021

Sunday, August 29, 2021
10:31 AM

- Biden administration not mandating COVID vaccines for White House staff, Psaki says
- https://www.breitbart.com/politics/2021/08/12/report-confidential-documents-reveal-pfizer-does-not-mandate-vaccines-for-employees/
- https://thehill.com/changing-america/well-being/prevention-cures/550394-nih-chief-says-he-is-not-requiring-his-employees
- https://sagaciousnewsnetwork.net/the-cdc-does-not-require-its-employees-to-be-vaccinated/
- modeRNA did not mandate it up until the FDA "approved it" so they reversed their policy https://www.bizjournals.com/boston/news/2021/08/20/moderna-covid-19-vaccine-staff-mandate.html

permalink parent save report block reply

From <https://patriots.win/p/12kFKzEivJ/dont-want-the-clotshot--/c/>

VAKS comments social media – note the need to "code" in response to FB censorship!

Keith McLaughlin, FB, UK

Well I'm not sure what it will take, if ever, to wake people up .
If losing a loved one in their sleep doesn't do it I don't know what will. My abbreviated experiences...
A close friend brother died in his sleep 3 weeks ago .. had had number 3 a week before to go to Spain without testing .. verdict "the heatwave" 🛐
A close friend had shingles a week after quack .. verdict stress
A close friend kept falling 10 days after quack .. fell ONTO the hot iron .. hospitalised.. tests found 'nothing' and told him he probably had an ear infection he believed them .
Close friend .. Bell's palsy .. but hey it was a coincidence.
My Ex's friend died within a week .. no no no .. he was stressed .
Neighbour 5 years clear of breast cancer .. now cancer in her liver.
TWO sisters went together for quack .. young women .. both had terrible bleeding ..BUT they did say they thought it was the quack.
Friends niece .. blood clot behind the eye a few days after .. looked like she'd been in a fight .. sight now blurred .. but yes they are now thinking it was number 2 .
Too many others to note .. general fatigue and lethargy are common .. periods irregular .. dear god we have no idea what the next years will hold for them🙂
For info … I'm in UK ..

<u>Keith Mc Laughlin</u>

Hi I'm from the Lake District UK.

My list of people gone and those not right is ever increasing.

3 dead a 56 yr old with massive brain bleed, 59 yr old Gillian Barre and one with exploded bowel.

Those not right include many with blood clots, pneumonia/fluid on lungs, severe sickness & dihorea, sepsis, 40 yr old with exploded bowel now with a bag, Guillian Barre, Heart Attacks, the list goes on with many issues including returning cancers and flu like symptoms several times in the juiced.

Hi Guys! I am a Nurse of 28 years...half my family didn't listen to me, but my parents and husband did. We went maskless and quack free since the beginning and have had no health issues. Meanwhile my sister has been quacked x3 and is 6 months pregnant. She is told that the baby is no longer growing anymore and they may induce. It's so frustrating that she let fear and propaganda rule her life the last almost 3 years. I am ashamed of the medical community and their ability to no longer critically think. My 85 yr old Father had to go into the hospital this past February due to fluid overload from Congestive Heart Failure and they said he tested + and that he would need R_______r[50] I fought with the pulmonologist and threatened to sue if they tried to quack him. Long story short he survived and was discharged despite them stating he was + and had to stay in the Hospital for 10 days. Fight for your family members! Question everything.and don't let them go Into the hospital alone if you can help it!!! BTW I have been following a Righteous MD (DM me for her

---

[50] Remdesivir, lethal prescription meds used "justify" use of pressurised oxygen to puncture lungs damaged by it.

info) since this all started and if it wasn't for her speaking out and her knowledge from interviewing Righteous Doctors my Father would have died in the Hospital. They would have killed him. Praying for all of you that suffered under the horror of this evil Globalist Scum!!!

By the first couple of months of 2021 my Mam had been x2 quacked. I'd begged her not to have any. By the April she was diagnosed with aggressive stage 4 cancer. Liver, bones. After showing initial improvements the specialist said the cancer was not acting like anything they'd seen before or responding as they'd normally expect. Spread to lymphatic system and her brain. As a family we didn't get the clarity of answers we should have. Mam passed away January this year 9 months after diagnosis. The most loving, caring and selfless beautiful mother. Just 74 years young. A life of good general health She should still be with us. The UK authorities, medical, political and those complicit in its delivery, they murdered my Mam and the loved ones of countless other families.

Jeannie Paice **August 24, 2022**

<u>osontSderp494uf58fa7fl6tgi8tol24hi19mcf51ho6ahg7iot mocmcc774</u> ·
Ths comes from a nurse who wants to stay anonymous
I'm a Nurse in the UK. I am anonymous because I don't want to be hunted by the hospital I work for (again - I have already stood up for the quack injured and been subjected to an 8 week investigation which resulted in them saying 'we do not dispute what it is you're saying' and received no sanctions).
Two staff members have had pulmonary embolisms and two staff on the neighbouring ward have had close relatives cardiac arrest, one died at the age of 30 two days after the

'boost' and one was successfully resuscitated, no older than 35. Loads of unusual and agrressive cancers emerging. We are checking people for blood clots more frequently and there are significantly more younger people on the stroke unit.

I have two friends that are suffering disability as a result of the quack, it's undeniably related and they tell me of more people they are aware of and the results are shocking. One of them sent me the details of a 24 year old, otherwise healthy with no past medical history, two weeks after the quack her parents found her dead in bed. 10 local people to my knowledge (might be more I am not aware of as they are never placed in the obituaries aged between 24-46 (46 was a mountain trekker so fit) that died suddenly or had a cardiac arrest. Two survivors and one has an hypoxic brain injury as it took 9 minutes to attempt resuscitation and not one person bothered to start before the ambulance arrived.

I worked on Covid for 2 years. 8 members of staff declined the quacks including one Dr. He said that at the start of the rollout he worked in ITU and saw too many people having brain haemorrhages and that's what put him off.

Without a frank conversation and further research these quacks should be halted. But no one wants to talk about it and they give them out to unsuspecting citizens who have faith in them. I have spent the last 18 months feeling completely heartbroken.

I could go on all day, I don't believe these quacks are safe for some, feels like roulette, a good game if you win, but if you lose it can be catastrophic.

Keith Mc Laughlin

Thank you for accepting me into this group. I have looked for a group like this for nearly a year now since my nightmare began. I am in the US. A year ago I was an active career woman with a bright future ahead of her. Now

I sit here broken and scared of my future with no idea what to do next. It all started with a sales meeting where my boss informed all of our department that he insisted that we get "quacked" and that we were all idiots for not doing it already. I expressed to him at this time my concerns and why I had chose all of the way up to that point not to do it. He still insisted. So off I went to go against my will to save the best job I had ever had and so I could continue to provide for my family. This was around the 1st of August 2021. Within a week my life was upside down. Tourette's like movements, migraines, fatigue to the max. By August 29th I was having full blown seizures and horrible stabbing pains all throughout my body along with uncontrollable shaking and all of my previous symptoms as well. At this point my employer is aware that the "quack" has done this to me and has let me officially start working from home with a promise to take care of me. Fast forward to the end of September when my employer decides to "let me go" through TEXT MESSAGE! Yes literally did not even have the decency to look me in the eyes when he did it. But let's move on. Fast forward to November and I am officially diagnosed with epilepsy and fibromyalgia. At this point money is running tight due to paying medical expenses out of pocket along with normal living expenses. Fast forward to January. Seizures are getting worse. I have a bad one and end up falling in my kitchen with concrete floors. MRI reveals my back is broken at the L5 and S1 and a disk is completely crushed. At this point I'm completely broke and on medicaid therefore waiting on an approval for the surgery takes time. It is also decided that it will be a complicated, lengthy surgery that they will have to coordinate 2 surgeons on. So, it took until June 7th to finally receive my spinal fusion surgery. Now, I walk with a cane constantly, I have partial paralysis in my left leg and horrific nerve pain throughout both legs. The doctors do not know if I will ever regain feeling. As for now, my seizures

and tremors seem to be under control with me taking 2 different medications twice a day. As for the pain I take gabapentin 3 times a day and tizanidine at night but I always still feel it, these meds just slightly dull it. I do have a lawyer actively trying to obtain my disability for me but no success as of yet. I do not know where to go from here or what resources might be available to me. Any help or suggestions would be so amazing and so appreciated. And if you read down this far, thank you for caring to read my story.
Copied and pasted

So...just came from hospital last night. My moms legs are black from the knees down because of blood clots. Her kidneys have shut down. She is intubated. In her will she stated she didn't want to be "kept alive" so the doctors are unhooking everything tonight. She has had 3 Quack shots. She lasted 32 minutes after everything was turned off.

Christina LaBette

tSpdsonreoga92lu9u625l4ou94325417h7f5f13665a7tou2 454f1518g1h ·
16months 2p
Recently was diagnosed with a blood clot in my leg, extending from my upper thigh to behind my knee. Just had chest MRI done to rule out PE. Was told no large PE but still possible to have a small clot in the lung. We are avoiding another CT scan as I've had well over 50 in the last 16 months. Now I have to have an ultrasound of my arm as I'm having symptoms of a clot there. I was also told by a holistic do that I have microclotting on top of all of the other stuff.
I have two testing appointments at Cleveland this week and next and I'm off all of my meds and utterly miserable. So for those that don't know I've been diagnosed with HMD

(hemiplegic migraine disorder is a rare neurological condition that mimics stroke), intractable migraines, complex migraines with aura, tachycardia, fibromyalgia, neuropathy, neurological deficits, pericarditis, pleural effusion, suspected MCAS (which did improve after allergist added on and increased meds), suspected POTS, possibly SFN, and we're still trying to figure out what is going on with my heart. Cardiologist also said she felt I have EDS. Rheumatologist said I'm having an overactive immune response, as well as an inflammatory response. I said give me something to stop it then. He suggested trying to get into a large university setting and finding a doctor who would admit me for an extended stay and getting them to run testing and med trials. This is just a nightmare.

I'm not giving up the fight, nor am I going to stop fighting for myself, and for those of us injured. I will continue spreading the word, trying to get help, and I pray for us all that we all stay strong and stick together so that we can get the help we truly need.

I've contacted all of my state representatives with no response, including members of congress, other state reps, and even tried reaching out to the WH. No luck. NIH sent me research links but we are well versed in most of that.

My dad said to me today to keep reaching out to them until they get annoyed with me. Keep calling, emailing, any way to contact because they will get so annoyed that they'll reach out. I hope this is true. I feel contacting the media is pointless as they won't do anything to help, let alone share our stories. I've given up on contacting P, CDC, Vaers, etc. They just keep giving me the run around and wanting me to start the paper process all over again when my doctors and myself have sent the documentation required and still no help, just a simple mailing each time.

VAX JAPAN DAILY MAIL JAN 2015

Why Japan banned MMR vaccine
by JENNY HOPE, Daily Mail
Japan stopped using the MMR vaccine seven years ago
- virtually the only developed nation to turn its back on
the jab.

Government health chiefs claim a four-year
experiment with it has had serious financial and
human costs.
Of the 3,969 medical compensation claims relating to
vaccines in the last 30 years, a quarter had been made
by those badly affected by the combined measles,
mumps and rubella vaccine, they say.
The triple jab was banned in Japan in 1993 after 1.8
million children had been given two types of MMR and
a record number developed non-viral meningitis and
other adverse reactions.
Official figures show there were three deaths while
eight children were left with permanent handicaps
ranging from damaged hearing and blindness to loss of
control of limbs.
The government reconsidered using MMR in 1999 but
decided it was safer to keep the ban and continue
using individual vaccines for measles, mumps and
rubella.
The British Department of Health said Japan had used
a type of MMR which included a strain of mumps
vaccine that had particular problems and was
discontinued in the UK because of safety concerns.
The Japanese government realised there was a problem
with MMR soon after its introduction in April 1989

when vaccination was compulsory. Parents who refused had to pay a small fine.

An analysis of vaccinations over a three-month period showed one in every 900 children was experiencing problems. This was over 2,000 times higher than the expected rate of one child in every 100,000 to 200,000.

The ministry switched to another MMR vaccine in October 1991 but the incidence was still high with one in 1,755 children affected. No separate record has been kept of claims involving autism.

Tests on the spinal fluid of 125 children affected were carried out to see if the vaccine had got into the children's nervous systems. They found one confirmed case and two further suspected cases.

In 1993, after a public outcry fuelled by worries over the flu vaccine, the government dropped the requirement for children to be vaccinated against measles or rubella.

Dr Hiroki Nakatani, director of the Infectious Disease Division at Japan's Ministry of Health and Welfare said that giving individual vaccines cost twice as much as MMR 'but we believe it is worth it'.

In some areas parents have to pay, while in others health authorities foot the bill.

However, he admitted the MMR scare has left its mark. With vaccination rates low, there have been measles outbreaks which have claimed 94 lives in the last five years.

(Author: This last paragraph is suspicious and leads to speculation regarding neglected and misdiagnosed

underlying conditions *or* *changes* *in* *population demographics.)*
Read   more: http://www.dailymail.co.uk/health/article-17509/Why-Japan-banned-MMR-vaccine.html#ixzz3wK7O0WbB

Follow   us: @MailOnline   on   Twitter | DailyMail   on Facebook

Postlude:

Another hero punished for saving lives.

Washington monument, anyone???

https://www.statesmanpost.com/doctor-indicted-for-allegedly-giving-fake-covid-vaccines-to-kids/

He gave saline, and not one of his patients died.

*If he accepted the "covid" bribes and bounty, and they try to charge him with fraud, I would accept that that was **essential** to keeping his cover and saving more lives, more children from the sudden, agonising death of the lethal, vascular destroying, circulation impairing*

APP triggering, spike protein producing, bestial human recombinant RNA.

The directors, facilitators and enablers of the producers of these bioweapons belong in High Security Prisons. Visited by the families of persons murdered by the high pressure vents and by the lethal bioweapons euphamistically and fraudulently called "Vaccines!

56,510 views Mar 6, 2023

Join The Conversation! | https://trialsitenews.com/ Physician-investigators at King Fahad University Hospital in Khobar, Eastern Province Saudi Arabia recently conducted a study, the largest of its kind, linking rare COVID-19 vaccine-related injuries and incidence of new onset of autoimmune disease, including systemic lupus erythematosus (SLE). The study team tapped into sources including the hospital's electronic medical record finding 31 patients with new onset post COVID-19 vaccine autoimmune diseases and a severe exacerbation of an existing disease including patients with connective tissue disorders, vasculitis, as well as neurologic diseases.

https://thetexan.news/houston-doctor-files-federal-lawsuit-against-fda-over-ivermectin-statements/

---

[i] In the West and Anglophone nations there is a strong tradition of making marriage proposals on the 14th of February each year...

[iii] Global diminution of respect for Americans may be an added bonus for hostiles. In allowing the bodies of American citizens to be sold to a foreign country, e.g., China, for dissection, experimentation, or covert DNA combo research, the psychological effect is diminution of respect, image of vulnerability; and given that, circumstantially, many of those bodies appear to come from "Potters field," i.e., the poor and homeless, this would further demote the image of America In the eyes of the less developed nations.
[iv] University of North Carolina
[v] William Shakespeare, Hamlet
[vi] https://pubmed.ncbi.nlm.nih.gov/32345113/ Data indicate that 82% of transgender individuals have considered killing themselves and 40% have attempted suicide, with suicidality highest among transgender youth.... 88% of that 82% are young, white and middle class.
[vii] https://williamsinstitute.law.ucla.edu/wp-content/uploads/Race-Ethnicity-Trans-Adults-US-Oct-2016.pdf

[viii] https://www.lifesitenews.com/news/toxic-by-design-researcher-explains-why-us-defense-depts-covid-vax-operation-shows-intent-to-harm/?utm_source=digest-prolife-2023-01-20&utm_medium=email

https://www.statesmanpost.com/pfizer-accused-of-manipulating-covid-vaccine-trial-data/?utm_placement=SPNews&clientId=merged-field-value

- Biden administration not mandating COVID vaccines for White House staff, Psaki says
  - https://www.breitbart.com/politics/2021/08/12/report-confidential-documents-reveal-pfizer-does-not-mandate-vaccines-for-employees/
  - https://thehill.com/changing-america/well-being/prevention-cures/550394-nih-chief-says-he-is-not-requiring-his-employees
  - https://sagaciousnewsnetwork.net/the-cdc-does-not-require-its-employees-to-be-vaccinated/
- ModeRNA did not mandate it up until the FDA "approved it" so they reversed their policy
  - https://www.bizjournals.com/boston/news/2021/08/20/moderna-covid-19-vaccine-staff-mandate.html

permalink parent save **report** block reply

https://www.youtube.com/watch?v=_f2WFFwBZPc
RNAse cross contamination

From <https://patriots.win/p/12kFKzEivJ/dont-want-the-clotshot--/c/>

https://alexberenson.substack.com/p/urgent-urgent-1-in-780-german-kids/comments

[ix] "Tribe of Cannibals: Operation Take Down America" is a revealing account of life in a "NY Gulag" an island on which a sinister psycho social experiment was conducted by Columbia U, Soros, UN, Democrat Party, etc., to examine the most effective ways to transform the USA

from a Constitutional Republic to a top down neo Feudal Corporate entity.

^x Encyclopedia Britannica

^{xi} Right again. Circa April 21st 2023 media announced that snake venom was used in some of the "vaccines" / bioweapons. Snake venom is generally associated with haemorrhage of intense bleeding, but there are a number of snakes whose venom is "thrombotic" or clot forming.

^{xii} https://medcraveonline.com › IPMRJ › transhumanism-the-big-fraud-towards-digital-slavery.htm

https://www.euvolution.com › prometheism-transhumanism-posthumanism › eugenics › why-nazis-
https://www.technology.org/2020/06/16/immortal-silicon-valley-top-transhumanist-projects-and-startups/